CONTENTS

Advance Praise for
Confessions of a Fat Cosmo Girl

"A true inspiration...Hazel Dixon-Cooper's book is an in-depth, honest, and eye-opening look at the diet industry...and is a must read for everyone who has ever considered a quick-fix weight-loss plan."

—**Craig & Jenny Dumnich**, Co-Founders of CraigandJennyD,
Fusion Performance Institute & Retreats Re-Imagined

"With humor and piercing insight into the diet culture, Hazel teaches us how to heal our relationship with food and with ourselves. We highly recommend this book as a guide to help anyone stop yo-yo dieting and learn how to listen to their body."

—**Thane & Cynthia Murphy**, Assuaged, Inc.

"Your life is about to change for the better. Hazel Dixon-Cooper shares her incredible journey and gives us the tools to defeat Inner Bitch, that self-sabotaging voice in our head. The Twenty-One-Day Challenge is brilliant. With every box you check off, you will feel stronger and more determined to succeed."

—**Tonya Reiman**, Body Language Expert, Behavioral Specialist,
and Author of *The Yes Factor*

"There's no shortcut or magic potion for maintaining good health. It's a journey (and) Hazel Dixon-Cooper depicts the multiple facets of that journey. This powerful book will cheer you on as you learn how to conquer every fear and defeat every nagging thought so you can achieve your wellness goal."

—**Denise N. Simpson**, Author of *Rejuvenate Your Health in 8 Simple Steps*

CONFESSIONS OF A FAT COSMO GIRL

HOW I LOST 122 POUNDS
& KEPT IT OFF & HOW YOU CAN TOO

HAZEL DIXON-COOPER

Post Hill
PRESS

Post Hill Press
New York • Nashville
posthillpress.com
Published in the United States of America
1 2 3 4 5 6 7 8 9 10

STOP KILLING YOURSELF

As I was writing this book, the world suffered through one of the most horrific pandemics in history. Even with our modern health care systems, medications, and scientific expertise, we were all vulnerable to a new threat to which no one was immune. The daily news reports and posts I read on social media reinforced how much our mindset matches our beliefs. People who refused to respect physical distancing and denied the danger posed by the virus caused only more damage. Denying the facts about the harm you're doing to your body with the foods you eat is just as dangerous. Being obese increased both the severity of COVID-19 and the chances of dying.[1]

During that time, I read countless posts and blogs and articles about how to raise immunity with proper nutrition and about the nutrient-rich foods found in a plant-based diet. Every piece of advice pointed to the simplest of actions: eat more vegetables, grains, and plant-based whole foods. Nothing is a 100 percent guarantee against illness. But keeping your body free of the toxins and chemicals found in processed foods while fueling it with food that boosts your well-being will always give you a better chance of living healthier and protecting yourself from any disease.

As a child, maybe you were told to clean your plate even though you were full. Perhaps you got a cookie as a reward or to soothe you when you skinned your knee. Perhaps you were told you "should" eat this and "shouldn't" eat that. Maybe you didn't get enough food or love and you ate to fill an emotional hole. Perhaps you're stuffing your face to stuff down the anger and helplessness you feel.

You might have been raised on fried food, fast food, or junk food and think you can't live without it. Maybe you were told that you inherited the family fat gene and there's nothing you can do to lose weight, or maybe you think that food is the only thing that can make you feel good. Forget it. These are just more excuses to keep you from becoming healthy.

I'm going to show you how I stopped automatically reaching for food and how you can recognize that nasty voice in your head for who and what she is and talk her down. I'll help you understand how to rewire the pathways that form unhealthy behavior patterns and create new, positive ones.

Maybe you have tried Weight Watchers, Jenny Craig, Nutrisystem, or any one of the hundreds of weight-loss programs on the market and were unsuccessful each time. Maybe you've tried joining a gym or watching online exercise videos and were as unsuccessful at sweating off what you ate that day as you were with the weight-loss programs. Perhaps you are considering bariatric surgery or have had it and are gaining back the pounds. Every ad, every weight-loss consultant, even your doctor has promised you an easy fix to your long-term food abuse. Forget it. There's no such thing.

The $80 billion weight-loss industry is designed to ensure you fail. You are obsessed with food, and they know it. They profit by keeping you obsessed. If you were healthy, they'd close their doors. So stop blaming yourself. All these miracle cures, including the big three—Weight Watchers, Nutrisystem, Jenny Craig—advertise long-term success. Yet, according to a study published by the National Institute of Health, losing 10 percent or more of your body weight and keeping it off for at least one year is considered the standard for "successful weight loss in obese individuals." After that time, the majority of people regained weight no matter what program they had tried.[2]

Further, the chances of keeping the weight off for five years or more is about 5 percent. This 95 percent long-term failure rate is what no commercial weight-loss program will tell you. This book will expose the propaganda you've heard from the weight-loss industry, from the ads on TV, and from medical and fitness professionals.[3]

You will learn:

- How the weight-loss industry keeps you fat.
- The truth about the feed-your-obsession snack foods they push you to buy.
- The diet-speak vocabulary that's designed to make you think getting healthy is a snap.
- The eat-the-foods-you-love story that leads you down the greasy path to illness, or worse.

You cannot eat Calorie-Rich and Processed foods (CRAP) and ever expect to kick the cravings. The weight-loss industry tricks you with portion control. Sure, if you eat less of anything you will lose weight. You will not lose your cravings for fat, carbs, and sugar. As soon as you're milked for all the money you can afford, you quit. Then, the weight piles on again because you still crave the junk and can no longer control yourself.

You gain back every pound and more, and then renew the mail-order meatloaf or head to a meeting for a dose of don't-worry-you-can-lose-it-again. Sure, you can. You will also gain back every pound because they all fail to teach you how to change your mindset. You can stay in this endless cycle until you're dead, which you will be if you don't flip off your fat switch for good. Or you can jump off the fat wagon and take responsibility for your health and your life. No one can do it for you.

No one could do it for me either, and believe me, I used every dodge in the book of self-deception. My pig-outs, cop-outs, and brain scuttle to avoid seeing the truth are all here. You'll recognize them because sneaking and cheating and lying are universal. I understand the panic you feel when you're anxious to lose, and the frustration when you repeatedly fail. I know what it feels like to hide food and lie to family, friends, doctors, and, worse, to myself. There isn't anything you have done that I haven't.

Feeling like a failure—sometimes desperate, sometimes defiant—I was always guilty because I knew how to lose weight but couldn't keep it off. I understand going to the biggest checker in the grocery line because you can't endure the side-eye from a cashier looking at your overloaded basket. Or cringing from a look the server at your favorite restaurant shoots you when bringing a huge plate of food. Knowing that others are quick to judge you by your size, thinking you're lazy because you can't lose the weight or a loser because you keep cycling through one weight-loss program after another, is humiliating.

I wrote this book because I understand how you feel. I know what it's like to be ashamed of the way you look and to feel so defeated that you use food to dull your emotional pain, just like drug addicts use heroin to dull theirs. I know what it's like to buy a package of Oreos one day, and then reach for it the next and wonder why there are only two or three cookies left.

I am going to show you how you can permanently change your attitude toward food. You will discover why your friends and family often sabotage you. You will understand how you can begin from where you are right now. You don't even have to believe in yourself. You just have to start. I ended my bingeing, guilt, and unhealthy eating by moving to a plant-based diet. It saved my life.

Most people don't wake up until their bodies are already damaged, or worse, they don't realize until it is too late that they are rotting from the inside out. Then they die. Don't let this be you.

CHAPTER 1

THE ELEPHANT IN THE ROOM

Hi Hazel,

I have an exciting lead. Cosmo is scouting out a new astrologer for the magazine. Are you interested? Let me know when you can!

The email from my publicist at Simon & Schuster appeared on my office computer, and for a moment, I froze. The news both thrilled and terrified me. At fifty pounds overweight, I was the anti *Cosmo* girl and, at that instant, would have given anything to be thin. As soon as that thought hit my brain, I panicked as I'd done so many times before. I flicked off the computer screen and headed for the company cafeteria.

Eating Anxiety

"The regular, Hazel?" the overweight server behind the counter asked.

"Yes." I was glad she was on duty because I knew I would get bigger portions if someone my size dished them out. She placed a huge apple fritter on a plate and handed it to me. I couldn't wait to dig in. Then, I got a cup of coffee with cream and sugar. Under any kind of stress, I automatically reached for something to eat like a drunk reaches for one more drink. Anything sugary, greasy, and calorie-laden was the temporary fix I used to dull the emotions I couldn't face.

Staring me right in my puffy cheeks was a chance to write the most well-known astrology column for the most successful women's magazine on the planet. What did I do? Rush for the worst thing I could eat, as always. I took my tray to a small table near a window that overlooked the patio and began to numb the excitement and fear I felt. There's a good reason we call it comfort food. For about thirty seconds, the mouthful of pastry and sweetened coffee warmed me, both physically and emotionally. But as soon as I swallowed the first bite, the glow faded, and I had to shove another forkful in my face, and then another and another until I was so stuffed that I couldn't feel anything but the food. After finishing the last bite, I justified the guilt I felt with the excuse that I would start dieting tomorrow. If you have done the same thing, you know that swearing off food is easiest when you're stuffed, and tomorrow is always the day.

As I sat there watching people outside walk by, a crazy thought flashed through my head. I didn't even have to talk to *Cosmo*. I was working full-time, writing a book, and caring for my family. No one would blame me for saying I didn't have the time to add another job to my schedule. In fact, no one would have to know. I hadn't told anyone yet. Not my family. Not my coworkers. Not my best friend. I could quietly decline this opportunity and just forget the whole thing, except I wanted to write that column. I'd been reading *Cosmopolitan* since I was a teenager. How could I not respond? The look, the confidence, the no-fear attitude that *Cosmo* represented was what I'd always wanted, but the one thing I could never pull together on a consistent basis.

Back at my desk, I spent the next four hours vacillating between fear and elation. Finally, I responded to my publicist who contacted the magazine and scheduled a telephone appointment with an associate editor for later in the day. Then I called my best friend and told her what was happening. I left out the part about how long it took me to pick up the phone, but hearing her enthusiasm helped me to feel better.

The editor was easy to talk with and explained that I would have to submit an audition column. She would send me samples of previous Bedside Astrologer columns via overnight mail so I could review the tone of the magazine. I had a week to write a piece for consideration. The whole conversation took about twenty minutes. A few days later, I submitted my audition material, and a day later, the editor called to offer me the job. My friends and family were excited for me, and I wanted to be overjoyed, but my self-sabotaging Inner Bitch reared her nasty head. If anyone saw what I looked like, I'd be dumped on my fat ass.

Wait, I thought. I'm in California, and the magazine is in New York. They don't know what size I am, and they don't have to find out. Besides, I can lose the weight fast.

Sure, I could have. But of course, I didn't.

Celebrating with a Binge

Cosmo hired me the Monday before Thanksgiving. Although that negative voice began to mumble in the back of my mind, I shut her up with one of every overweight person's go-to excuses.

I deserve to celebrate.

So, instead of jumping off the fat wagon, I fell face first into the mindless pig-out of a holiday binge. By seven o'clock in the morning on Thanksgiving Day, I had poured my second cup of coffee with cream and sugar and sampled the dried fruit I had chopped for the dressing.

How harmful are a few pieces of fruit? This is my breakfast.

The food fog had descended, and the vow I had made a few days before vanished.

With few exceptions, I'd been cooking Thanksgiving for almost thirty years for anyone who wanted to show up to celebrate. That tradition had started several years before I was married, when two friends and I decided one year that we would rather celebrate together than travel to be with our respective families. After I got married, our family get-togethers again morphed into friends-only celebrations. My dinners were strictly traditional—turkey, stuffing, potatoes, gravy, a couple of side dishes, and desserts. My daughter liked to help me prepare dinner, and my husband liked to sample every dish.

Our best friends and their daughter arrived first.

"Congratulations!" My friend hugged me with one arm, and then handed me a platter of homemade cookies.

"I'm so excited for you," another friend said. "I love *Cosmo*." She set a small Crock-Pot full of chili dip on the counter as I emptied a family-size bag of corn chips into a bowl.

That year we hosted nine, and by the time the last couple walked in with a vegetable tray, the little restraint I had managed to have while cooking evaporated. It made no difference that the calorie intake from my before-dinner dinner was enough for the day, or that I had sworn to eat healthier, or that I wasn't even hungry. When the feast was ready, I attacked the food as if I were starving.

At the table, I savored every bite I could pack into my belly. Later, I ate my way through a variety of desserts. A slice of pie. A sliver of cake. A couple of cookies. Stuffed as tight as the turkey we had just devoured, I staggered through the rest of the evening in a stupor.

My friends had been thrilled for me. They had also helped me fail. *Eat, Haze. You can start your diet on Monday.* Of course, I agreed. I had much to celebrate and deserved every bite. Best of all, Monday was four days away. By bedtime, I had rationalized that I really hadn't eaten that much. The next morning, I awoke bloated and sluggish. My head ached. I had a food hangover and looked like hell. The self-defeating noise in my brain, on the other hand, was having a field day. *How could you be so damn stupid? You are such a loser.* She blasted me with every nasty name in the book of self-criticism.

I dressed, made coffee, and went straight to my desk to work on my first column. There I sat, as bleary-eyed as if I had spent all night at the neighborhood bar. I wrote horoscope predictions such as, "Single? Venus sparks your sexual fire. A passing glance ignites a cutie's passion. Attached? Your libido gets a feisty fuel injection. Stock up on oysters and vitamins—he'll need both to keep up with you." By then, the only thing igniting my passion was the thought of leftovers. Before long, I was rummaging through the fridge.

My new diet day was still a long weekend away, and I spent the next three days using my body as a garbage disposal for the last remnants of dinner, dessert, and junk food. All had to go before I could start fresh with a perfect new lifestyle of healthy eating. That wasn't the first time I had gorged myself on everything I could find in preparation for the next diet. Maybe you have done the same thing.

That urge to stuff yourself before your next attempt to lose weight is real. The fear of forever giving up the fattening foods you love and having to live on carrot sticks and lettuce for the rest of your life can trigger a binge of mindless eating. Instead of seeing a chance to get healthy, you view the next diet as a way to punish yourself because you're overweight. All that does is open the door for your Inner Bitch to start berating you, and put you in danger of giving up before you get started, which is exactly what happened to me. By Monday morning, I had conveniently forgotten my promise to myself, and the worst wasn't even in sight.

The holiday season flew by in a blur of deadlines, work, and shopping, all planned around food. After-work wine and appetizers, and then a deli sandwich on the way home. Saturday shopping and a dessert reward from my favorite bakery. Lunches with friends. Holiday parties. The company celebration was always a giant buffet, and I grazed through the line all evening. And I wasn't the only one bingeing before swearing to start fresh in the new year. Facebook was full of photos of people at various gatherings, sitting behind plates piled with food. Their posts were all a similar version of how they were feasting before facing the famine of another resolution to lose weight.

Between Christmas and New Year's, several of my coworkers brought their leftover candy and desserts from home because they were smart enough to not want the stuff around the house. Not me. I didn't share. I did munch all day.

Thinking that your future is one of deprivation is a destructive fantasy, just the same as thinking eating less calories of fattening foods will help you long term. If you stay under a certain calorie limit for your size, you can eat nothing but Snickers bars and lose weight, but you will not be healthy and you certainly won't lose your cravings for sugar. That's what the weight-loss industry counts on and why the majority of people who try commercial diets don't succeed.

Instead of approaching a diet like it is a prison sentence, think about what you are trying to accomplish. Don't wait for the right time, or after the next celebration, or until you have a serious health scare, as I did when I was diagnosed with coronary artery disease. Start saving your life now. Aim for steady improvement instead of instant gratification. One step. One bite. One day at a time.

Hiding the Junk

Every overweight person has a secret stash of junk food. I had several. Although I took the candy dish off my desk at work, I simply transferred the sweets to the back of the bottom drawer. I buried a family-size bag of Peanut M&Ms and box of Junior Mints under the maps and assorted change in the car's console. My purse always held a few pieces of whatever I currently happened to crave.

In my home office, a cache of mini candy bars lay in a box on the floor under my desk. The sugar high got me through the late-night cram sessions to meet my deadlines. That was my excuse. The truth was that I was in the middle of a mindless feeding frenzy.

Lies are easier to tell yourself when there are no witnesses. I used phrases such as *borderline diabetic* and *high-normal blood pressure* as euphemisms to avoid the truth about how I was ruining my health. I justified hiding food because I didn't want to have to listen to another lecture, well-meant or not. What I really didn't want was to have to be accountable for what I was doing to my body and my health. So I became a stealth eater and nearly the size of a stealth bomber. When the stash under my desk was empty, I headed to the kitchen and raided the pantry.

While shopping for groceries, I would buy a candy bar and eat it on the way home. I've seen other overweight people eat single-serving bags of potato chips or cookies as they grocery shop, and then pay for the empty bag at the checkout counter. I always went to a checker who was bigger than me because I felt comfortable knowing he or she would not think about the crap loaded in my cart. Regardless of whether the normal-size checkers may or may not have judged me, I judged myself.

I lied to myself that I was still dieting and that these daily slips didn't mean that much. Even when I was a member of Weight Watchers, and bought its boxes of snack bars, I was likely to eat at least one box that day, sometimes right after the meeting as I was completing my errands before going home. That's why I always bought several.

You may be doing the same sneaky eating. You hide the amount of worthless junk you consume from your family and friends and have at least one secret stash, one you wouldn't share even in the apocalypse. Maybe just reading my confession has made you hungry, and you are reaching for whatever floats your personal food-Titanic. I know. I've done that too.

Some days I would panic because, for a moment, I'd wake up and see the damage I was doing. Then, just as I had done a thousand times before, I'd swear off food. For a couple of days or a week, I would lay off the junk, but never long enough to make a real difference.

Like a drunk in a blackout, I hadn't a clue how much food I shoved in my face over the holidays. When I reluctantly stepped on the scales at the end of the year, I had gained almost fifteen pounds. Even when handed the opportunity of my dreams, I was still destroying my life with food. Writing for *Cosmo* hadn't thrilled me or shamed me enough to stop overeating. Instead of acknowledging the elephant in the room, I had become the elephant.

CHAPTER 2

MIND GAMES

You choose to live a healthier lifestyle. The decision to do so is not easy, and sticking to it takes a consistent, committed effort. Often, you're met with all kinds of resistance or skepticism from your family and friends, but none is more sabotaging than that voice in your own head.

Meet Inner Bitch

She is the negative voice that never stops yapping. Whether berating you with cruel comments about your shortcomings, or quietly encouraging you to fail by pretending to be your best friend, this bitch is tricky, and she will kill you if she can.

No matter how successful you are at managing your job or your home, no matter how good a parent or friend you are, she's always spewing a steady stream of abuse. *You're a failure. You're stupid. You never do anything right.* That's when she's easy to recognize. She's even more deadly when she pretends to be on your side. One day, she spews venom, and the next day or next hour, all you hear is a quiet, friendly voice giving you all kinds of seemingly rational excuses to give up. My Inner Bitch is as friendly as she is mean. *This is a special occasion. Go ahead and splurge. You deserve a treat.* That's how dangerous and destructive she can be. She even whispers that it's okay to start tomorrow or next week or next month, but procrastination can be deadly. Stalling about getting serious with your health causes stress, which only adds to the strain your body is under from being overweight. Procrastination has been linked to physical problems: from poor sleep, to digestive disorders, to more susceptibility to colds and the flu, to high blood pressure, and heart disease. All the while, you're fueling more self-critical thoughts, which only cause more stress. Ignoring my own expanding size and climbing blood pressure escalated my health issues from permanently aching joints to cardiovascular disease.

One reason Inner Bitch keeps harping at you is that your brain is wired for routine. Just like your morning routine and your mindless eating habits, the endless self-criticisms running through your head have become automatic. You overeat. Bitch berates you. You feel bad. You overeat. The excuses you use work the same way. You overeat. Bitch rationalizes the binge. You feel justified. You overeat. Until you learn how to shift your thinking to take away her power, you can't change.

This constant stream of no-win chatter is called distorted thinking, and it has many forms.

A woman I talked to had lost and regained more than one hundred pounds multiple times. One of her distorted thinking patterns was that she was either obsessive about counting every calorie and measuring every ounce of food she ate, or she just tried to "watch" what she ate, which always led to gaining again.

Another way she avoided the truth was to try to take the focus off her challenges by changing the subject. She would jump to discussing the latest book or diet that she had found on the internet.

She used her and her husband's preference for eating out as a way to justify a pattern of overeating. Our conversations were like playing mental ping-pong. Every question I asked was deflected with an excuse. Every goal she set was postponed. The reasons varied from guests dropping by, to a birthday celebration, to being too stressed to cook dinner and either eating out or relying on prepackaged foods. One day, she told me that she had finally realized that she didn't have the fat switch I talk about. "I was born without that switch, so there's nothing I can turn off," she said. This seemed to be the ideal excuse to give up. She had been born without the ability to control herself. Not her fault. The fact that she had succeeded several times didn't count. The fact that she knew how to lose weight didn't count. The only voice she heard and believed was her own destructive Inner Bitch.

You think because you've regained weight that you will never be able to keep it off regardless of what you do. Worse, you may think you don't deserve to be healthy because you struggle. You may blame others for your low self-esteem. None of these self-berating ideas do anything but give you an excuse to keep eating. For years, I lost every battle because I wrongly believed that voice in my head. Inner Bitch is the worst critic we have. She holds us back, destroys our self-esteem, and makes us think we cannot win no matter what we do. She clouds our thinking when it comes to spotting the harm we let others do to us.

Recognize the Voices of Sabotage

When you decide to take control of your life and your health, those changes can make the people close to you very uncomfortable. Making significant changes in your life means at least some adjustments in theirs, and they often will respond to your decisions with their own distorted thinking patterns.

You tell your friend, hoping she will support your effort. Instead, she says, "Again? I hope it works this time."

You tell your spouse you are committed to succeeding, and he or she might say, "I love you just the way you are," or snap, "How much will it cost this time?"

Your mother or brother or best friend prepares your favorite dessert to celebrate your first ten-pound loss and rationalizes, "You can't starve yourself all the time."

If you've heard comments like these, you aren't alone. A Stanford University School of Medicine study showed that more than 75 percent of women never or rarely experienced support from family and friends when trying to lose weight.[1]

Sharing your goal to live a healthier lifestyle is often threatening to others. *If you lose a lot of weight, you might leave me. If you get thin, you might look better than I do. If you can do this, what will you decide to do next?* Their reactions can be as grounded in distorted thinking as yours.

You drop the French dip in favor of grilled vegetables. Your friend, who has just ordered the all-you-can-eat pasta, looks at you as if you are betraying her because she may feel pressured to start shedding some pounds. You pass on the chocolate lava cake, and she says, "Well, if you aren't having dessert, I guess I shouldn't either." Your choices have triggered her negative self-talk. She may be blaming you for making her feel guilty about her own lifestyle. Those feelings have nothing to do with you. That's her distorted thinking process.

When you are no longer the fat friend that makes the skinny friend look even smaller, their insecurity and jealousy can damage the relationship. A woman I'd been friends with for decades acted as if she didn't notice my shrinking body. I'd been fighting my weight for years, while she never gained a pound. We lived in different cities and saw each other about once a month. When we celebrated each other's birthday or a holiday, she always brought her camera to record the occasion. I hated to have my picture taken and always had an expression that was more cringe than smile. As my weight loss became noticeable, she stopped bringing her camera. Maybe my success threatened her self-esteem.

An overweight colleague with whom I often had lunch began calling me Skinny Minnie almost the moment I told her I was determined to lose and keep the weight off. Asking her to stop did no good.

"I'm just joking," she insisted.

When you are no longer a part of a feeding-frenzy duo, your co-dependent friend feels threatened. When you trash your family's fat-gene excuse by losing weight, they feel threatened. Sound familiar? Your success may remind others of their failures. They see your hard work and progress, and then their Inner Bitch begins to beat them up. They may act as if they're on your side, but unconsciously or not, they won't relax until you fail again.

No matter what you hear from other people, you are not responsible for what they may think or feel about your choice to get healthy.

Don't Compromise

You've given in when everyone goes for pizza. You've shared the dessert so your friend won't feel bad. You've let your spouse's fears stop you. Compromising and yielding to others' expectations has done nothing but harm you.

Getting your spouse to help instead of hinder you is important. Chances are, if you're overweight, so is your partner, but they may not be ready to commit to changing what they eat. Don't let that stop you. If they live in your house and eat at your table, they should be on board. When you cook healthier meals, they will eat better. When you clear out the junk food, they can't eat it either.

Of course, you can continue to eat anything anyone shoves your way to avoid conflict and appease those around you. Keep that attitude and you could turn into an insulin-shooting diabetic stumbling around on your last three toes, eat yourself into a case of dementia, or be diagnosed with late-stage cancer because the fat hid the tumor. This self-sabotaging behavior can shove you right onto center stage at your own funeral.

No is a powerful word. Say it. Mean it.

- Be brief. You might be surprised at how a straightforward, "No, thank you," without further explanation can work.
- Stall. If it's hard for you to come right out and say no, then say something like, "Looks delicious, but I'm stuffed," or "Maybe later."
- Don't give in. When dealing with a pushy person who keeps insisting on just one more bite or one extra serving, keep repeating your no.

Often, we think refusing to do what another person wants means an argument. Fear of confrontation stopped me many times. I didn't want to rock the boat, so I didn't stand up for myself. After I finally began to say no, I discovered that usually nothing happens. Most of your tribe won't care if you don't have a second helping or eat dessert. They're conditioned to push food on you because, until now, you've always given in. They are also just as conditioned to eat too much of the wrong foods as you are. By choosing to change how you eat, you're disrupting the pattern, which may cause a bump. But once they realize you are serious, those who care about you will accept your choice. If they don't, then it's time for a change.

The friend who stopped taking photos at our get-togethers ignored my progress. She still expected me to share a double-size dessert with her and shot me oh-how-boring looks when I ordered salad instead of the fattening meals I used to eat. That opened the door for other, more serious issues that had always been wrong with our relationship—ones I had ignored because I was reluctant to disagree. Finally, I chose to end the relationship. At the time, I felt terrible. I also felt as if a proverbial ton of bricks had fallen off my shoulders.

As I began to consistently lose weight, the coworker I regularly ate lunch with distanced herself from me. Although we sometimes still ended up in the cafeteria at the same time and occasionally sat together, she found a new lunch partner.

Redefining some of your relationships will be painful. However, you must put yourself first. You might get a pout from your sister or lose an eating buddy at work, but isn't that better than destroying your health or losing your life? If you want to be healthy, you must take charge of what you eat. Don't ever apologize.

Listen to Your Body

Early on a Saturday morning, as I sat in my car in the parking lot of the neighborhood supermarket checking my grocery list, I saw an obese woman—who was carrying a box of pastries—shuffle out of the store. I watched as she slowly walked to her car and squeezed behind the wheel. As soon as she closed the door, she lifted the lid of the box, chose a doughnut, took one bite out of it, and then put the rest back in the box. I knew that before she arrived at home, the first doughnut would be history. Maybe she'd had a bad week at work and told herself she deserved a treat. Maybe she'd had a great week and told herself the same thing. Whatever the excuse she might have used, her behavior reminded me of how often I had done the same thing.

Whether you tell yourself you deserve to splurge or you just don't care or that food is the only pleasure you have, you're motivated by self-destruction, and the real reasons are guilt and shame. Every restriction you've placed on yourself is cut. Every rule is broken. Nothing matters but the sensation of the next bite and the next and the one after that until you're sick from the sheer volume. I've eaten until I've cried with frustration about what I was doing to myself. I've eaten because I was angry that I couldn't stick to a diet program and knew logically that I was going to gain every pound back but also knew emotionally that I couldn't stop. The cycle of bingeing and dieting is a downward spiral of using food as a weapon against emotions you can't control and feeling guilty that you're inflicting pain on yourself by eating nonstop. You eat when you're not hungry and don't stop when your body has had enough.

Binges are a way to say "go to hell" to your family or friends or the world because you can't say it aloud. They're a temporary way to numb the pain of a bad situation from the past and to stop feeling guilty over something you couldn't change or didn't have responsibility for in the first place. Binges are fueled by Inner Bitch, the voice that does nothing but lie to you. Whether she tells you that you're the worst person on the planet so go ahead and eat yourself to death or urges you to soothe yourself with another plateful of food, her aim is to destroy you.

You can't prevent other people from emotionally hurting you. But you can stop thinking that somehow you deserve the mean things they say or do. You can stop feeling you should have had the brains or the strength or the knowledge to outwit or fight whoever hurt you. You can stop punishing yourself with food.

Learning how to listen to your body instead of your head takes practice. Knowing when enough is enough means staying in the present moment. When you don't, the idea of what is enough keeps running ahead of you like the dangling carrot. I've had food binges where I've eaten bags of mini candy bars and fistfuls of potato chips or cookies. I've eaten huge dinners until I could barely breathe, and then gone back for more the instant that sick, crammed-full feeling subsided.

Once I began to look at food as fuel instead of using it as sedation to dull my emotions, I began to binge less. Once I began to learn that I could never eat enough to feel good about myself, I started to realize how I had used food as a shield against everything I disliked about my life. Although it took some health scares before I finally got the message that I could change, that doesn't have to happen to you. I learned that enough is not something you can eat or touch or buy. Enough is inside you. You are the only one who can discover that for yourself. You have to do the work. I can't do it for you. What I can do is remind you that you can succeed. Your body wants to be healthy. You deserve to be happy. You are as good as anyone else on this planet, and no one has the right to make you feel bad about yourself. Not even you.

CHAPTER 3

CHANGE BEGINS IN YOUR HEAD, NOT ON YOUR PLATE

You probably picked up this book because you're looking for another quick fix to losing those extra pounds your body has hauled around for years or decades. You're the woman who believes every negative thought crowding her head and who can't look herself in the eye in the bathroom mirror. I know who you are because I was no different. For twenty years, I tried everything from Weight Watchers to South Beach to SlimFast in an endless cycle of yo-yo dieting. On each downward swing, I lost fewer pounds while gaining more and more on the upswing.

Outwardly, I blamed my food addiction on everything from stress to being too tired to cook. I told myself I was an emotional eater. Good days, bad days, every day, I found an excuse to eat. Friday nights at my house were always either fast food or dinner out. My excuse for that was because no one should have to cook after a hard week at work. Inside, I was fighting a losing battle with Inner Bitch. Only a diagnosis of coronary heart disease could get my attention. Even then, the first thing I had to do was clear my mind of a running dialogue of self-sabotage.

Revise Your Mindset

Before you can take back control of your health and your life, you have to rescue your mind. Just as you're going to learn how to clean the toxins out of your body, you're going to learn how to begin to clear away the emotional poison that's swirling through your brain.

We all know how to lose weight. Eat less junk, processed, and fast food. Eat more vegetables, whole grains, and other plant-based foods. Move more. That is a simple formula. So why is it so hard to do? For one, you are addicted to fat, carbs, and sugar, and the weight-loss industry does nothing to help you kick that habit. More importantly, whether you learned that food was either a reward or a comfort in childhood, you've been conditioned to reach for food as an emotional crutch every time you're stressed, anxious, angry, or happy. You've become addicted to the temporary feel-good fix of feeling stuffed.

If you can suffer through Weight Watchers' points, Nutrisystem's food, Jenny Craig's price, or any other weight-loss plan—and pay hundreds or thousands of dollars for programs and products that have not worked for you—you already have the discipline to do it for yourself without the cost, the hype, or the repeated failures.

Pay Attention

We've all heard the word mindful, but what does mindfulness mean? Jon Kabat-Zinn, PhD, at the University of Massachusetts Medical School says, "Mindfulness is awareness that arises through paying attention, on purpose, in the present moment, non-judgmentally. It's about knowing what is on your mind."[1]

Being aware of your actions keeps your body and brain in sync. Instead of walking around on autopilot, you are alert to what you're doing right now. When applied to your eating habits, listening to your body's signals and being aware of your emotions can help you separate physical hunger from emotional hunger. Your body will tell you when it's hungry, and that's a lot less often than when you stuff it with anything remotely resembling food.

Focus on Eating, Not Multitasking

How many times have you answered texts, watched TV, or scrolled through Facebook or Instagram while eating? How many times have you eaten while walking around the house or searching for something on your desk or in the car? These behaviors totally distract your brain from the fact that you are eating, and you end up doing the three-minute cram. You barely taste your food and lose track of how much you eat. Mindful eating means paying attention to when and where you eat, as well as what and how much you consume.

- Turn off the technology. Chances are great that both your world and the planet will not fall apart without your constant vigilance.
- Sit down at the table and focus on your meal—with or without family or friends. You're retraining your brain to develop healthy habits and eliminating the signals that tell your mind it's okay to eat anywhere while doing anything.
- Eat slowly. We all gulp our food when we're in a hurry. But that too often becomes a habit even when we have plenty of

time for a leisurely meal. Shoveling food down your throat doesn't give your brain time to catch up with your body. If you're in a rush or have only a thirty-minute lunch break, eat half your meal and save the other half for later. Your body takes about twenty minutes to tell your brain it's full. When you have your brain on speed-chew, you can't hear your body's signals.

Trade Comfort for Nourishment

Comfort food. Think about that term. The purpose of food is to keep your body alive and healthy. That's it. Your mind may need comforting, but your body does not need comfort food. Ask yourself what comforts you other than food. Make a list of alternatives you can do other than eat when your emotional hunger flares. Here are some suggestions:

- Try an online exercise class.
- Hug someone.
- Call or text someone who supports you.
- Walk the dog. Play with the cat. Ride your horse. Have fun with your pets.
- Garden. Go to the nursery and buy a plant or herb garden.
- Walk with a friend, even if you're in different neighborhoods or towns. Arrange a time, and then talk on your cell phones while walking.
- Get a foot massage or give yourself one.
- Read a book or magazine.
- Play games that will get you off the couch.
- Reward yourself for not eating with a nonfood gift.

Think of more distractions that can help you to stop mindlessly reaching for food to try and fill your emotional needs.

Defeat Inner Bitch

A very effective exercise in keeping Inner Bitch quiet is to simply talk back. When you verbalize her nasty criticisms, and then answer with positive statements, you begin to recognize her slurs for the lies they are. You may discover who first planted those lies in your mind and when that occurred.

Next time you hear that negative voice say something like *you can't do anything right,* answer in the first person. You might start by saying, "That's a broad statement, bitch. I do a lot of things right. Here are a few to remind you." Then think about what you do and have done that contradicts these lies and tell her about them. Lisa Firestone, PhD, is a clinical psychologist and the Director of Research and Education for the Glendon Association. She explains that speaking aloud or writing down this dialogue "will help you see these thoughts as an alien point of view and not as true statements."[2]

If you're like I was, you may walk around talking to yourself for a long time until the voice begins to fade into the background. Fielding Inner Bitch's nasty criticism is like playing tennis. Every time you hit the ball across the net, she smashes another one at your head. Keep talking. You're learning to look objectively at these lies and see how irrational they really are. You may also recognize the human voice behind the one in your head.

Swear if you need to. Yelling works too. I've done both many times. Hearing your own angry voice standing up for yourself can boost your self-confidence in learning how to recognize her sabotage.

Recovering your true self requires stepping into the past to examine where and when you first heard those negative comments and who said them. Whether you were intentionally hurt or absorbed your family's dysfunction, you may be playing a role that someone else has defined for you. Only you can define who you are.

Recognize Your Limiting Beliefs

Limiting beliefs are the hurtful comments you overheard or were told in childhood that sabotage your motivation and keep you from reaching your goals. Inner Bitch exists to keep them looping through your brain. These false ideas lead to distorted thinking.

Maybe a sibling put you down, and then excused their bad behavior with, "Just kidding." You may grow up thinking that it's okay to let other people disrespect you or make cruel jokes at your expense because they, too, are just kidding. Even if you recognize this ugly behavior for what it is, you might be unable to stand up for yourself. Instead, you reach for food as a way to forget or comfort yourself. What you're really doing is eating your anger at both the people who talk down to you and yourself for not being able to confront them.

Maybe one or both of your parents criticized you "for your own good." Maybe Mom and Dad, or whoever your caregivers were, thought they were helping you. Maybe they were being callous. Whatever the reason, you've grown up with a distorted view of yourself.

Perhaps you brush off compliments because, deep down, you think you don't deserve them. *No one could possibly have anything good to say about me.* Everything in your head that isn't helping you move forward into health is a distortion that someone put there when you were a child. As an adult, you carry these memories, sometimes buried deep within your mind. Your limiting beliefs often act like magnets that attract the same types of self-sabotage into your life today. Limiting beliefs are hardwired into your brain. They make you feel worthless and seem so true because of the ongoing self-sabotage you create.

Your beliefs create your thoughts.

Your thoughts create your feelings.

Your feelings create your actions.

Your actions create your results.[3]

When you believe something about yourself, you filter everything through that belief. When limiting beliefs are running the show, you're creating a no-win situation.

These patterns aren't random. Your brain is like a computer, sorting and processing the information you take in through your senses and experiences. At the base of your brainstem is a bundle of nerves called the reticular activating system. This system takes what you believe and finds information to validate that belief. In other words, if you think you're bad at managing money, you probably are. If you think you'll never lose weight permanently, you probably won't. On the flip side, with intention, this filtering system can be reprogrammed. It works kind of like the law of attraction. What you expect to get, you attract. Say you buy a red car. Suddenly, you seem to see red cars everywhere you go. Your brain is zeroing in on finding as many red cars as it can.[4]

So if you believe you aren't capable or that you're bad or stupid or any other negative assumption, your brain finds all kinds of evidence to prove it to you.

Limiting belief: *I'm such a loser.*

Supporting reasons or distorted thinking: *I overate because I was too tired to cook, ordered a pizza, and couldn't resist the pan-size chocolate chip cookie. Now, I'm back to square one, so I might as well just keep eating.*

New positive belief: *I am not a loser.*

Supporting reasons: *I made one mistake at one meal. I've lost (X) pounds. I've eaten well for (X) days.*

Pick one of your most critical beliefs and write it down. Next, write down two or three reasons for that belief. Then, write a new, positive belief that contradicts the old, false one. At first, you might not believe this positive statement. That's okay. At first, you don't have to believe them. Just do the exercise.

For the next twenty-one days, consciously look for signs that confirm your new self-supporting belief. Write these down and review them every day for a few minutes. The longer you do this, the stronger your new belief will become.

We all have limiting beliefs and are full of distorted thinking patterns. So don't be surprised or discouraged when you hear Inner Bitch muttering others while you're working on the first one. Write those down too, along with a positive statement that disproves each one she spews. Be patient with yourself. You're aiming for consistency that leads to permanent change, not another quick fix.

Create Your Future

What if you could travel into your personal future? You might not have a time machine, but you do have an imagination, so let's take a trip to the future you.

Write down "I am (your age today + ten) years old." Describe exactly how you envision your future self. How do you want to look and feel? What will your home be like? Think about your friends, your job, education, romantic life, and family. Write down everything you want your future life to be. Don't rush. Take time to create a solid image before you go to the next step.

Now, imagine that your future self comes to visit. She looks just as you imagined and has the life you've described above. What advice would she give you to put you on the path to becoming her? Write down everything she tells you. Do not edit, criticize, or set any limitations. Don't let Inner Bitch derail you. Your older self is here to help you. She will tell you the truth without hurting you. Then make a list of the steps you can start taking today to create the future you want.

Next, imagine a dark, dirt road with deep ruts left by decades of cars traveling over it and a new, clean, well-lit road that runs beside the old one. The new one took a lot of work to create. The old one, although overgrown with weeds, is still there. The distorted thoughts that make you feel bad about yourself are like the old road. You will have to work at creating a new path, but you can do it. Doing this exercise helps you to actually create new, positive neuro pathways in your brain that can override the distortions and false beliefs you've been conditioned to accept.

Change takes courage and consistency. Doing these exercises might make you feel uncomfortable at first, but with practice, your confident voice will become stronger, and Inner Bitch's will fade.

CHAPTER 4

THE SHAME GAME

Every obese person has felt the sting of a disapproving look. We've all cringed at the thought of squeezing into a booth at a restaurant or been hyper-aware that our butt is hanging over the sides of the chair we hope doesn't collapse under our weight. No matter how we may pretend we didn't hear or see other people's nasty comments and disgusted looks, their reactions hurt. The shame others impose on you gets internalized, which only reinforces your own shame and may exacerbate your distorted thinking.

Recognize the Faces of Shame

Ever walked, head down, through the grocery store, thinking that everyone was judging you by the food in your cart? Have you glared right back at someone who stared at that carton of ice cream in your hand? Have you stood behind your friends in a group photo or used humor to put yourself down before anyone else could? You aren't alone.

Overweight people have a cast of characters living in their heads, and all perform on command for our personal Inner

Bitch. No matter the emotion or the scene, she uses shame to direct the action.

Little Girl & Good Guy

With their passive smiles and stooped shoulders, Little Girl and Good Guy are desperate to fade into the background. They are the floating heads trying to hide in the back row of any photo. You may find them sitting in the back row at an event or in the corner at a party. Little Girl wants to be thought of as a good person so she tries hard to appear cheerful and be helpful, deluding herself that if she's a really good girl, others won't judge her by her weight.

When eating out, both may arrive early and slide into the corner of a booth. Embarrassed to order the ribs and beans or steak and loaded potato she really wants, Little Girl orders a salad and diet soda. Then, because she is still emotionally hungry, she swings by the drive-thru on her way home. I can't tell you how many times I played this part. I'd order the salad, or whatever diet plate the restaurant offered, and then head straight for a sack of tacos at the drive-thru. Good Guy might eat more in public, but chances are he will also pick up more food on his way home.

Little Girl and Good Guy face their shame by either trying to disappear or be so pleasant that others won't care how big they are. They're desperate to be accepted. These people will often go out of their way to help others. They might be the friend who always offers to drive or the sales clerk who goes out of their way to help or the person who's always first to respond in a crisis. They have an abundance of compassion for everyone but themselves.

The Co-Conspirator

A Co-conspirator tries to make you a partner in her addiction. She's the one who sees you watching her place three huge French bread pizzas in her shopping cart and is compelled to justify herself. "These are on sale," she might say. "You can freeze them." Sure. You and she both know those pizzas won't last long enough to place in the freezer. That's because you've done the same thing. Me too.

Co-conspirators seek validation for their destructive behavior. These are friends or family members who reinforce each other's overeating with mutual reassurance that they deserve to be bad. Translation: when you need a pig-out, you feel protected when with another person you trust not to judge you—like the couple I saw at the grocery store who were buying potatoes. He had selected a huge baking potato, about twice the size of a standard potato and easily large enough for two people. As he began to put it in the grocery cart, she asked him, "Should we get one or two?" He nodded and asked her to pick another one. She could have been thinking they could have one that night and one later in the week, but I doubt it. I've been there and done that too.

The Joker

The Joker is a put-down artist and always the butt of their own jokes. I saw an obese young man at the gym who wore a t-shirt with *Drink Until You Want Me* printed across the front. Although he grinned at anyone who made eye contact, beneath that jolly façade, I'm sure his Inner Bastard was shouting *you fat loser*.

I, too, made lame attempts at humor to cover my embarrassment about my size. "I thought I'd worked my ass off," I'd tell my friends anytime I felt uncomfortable. "Unfortunately, when I looked in the mirror this morning, it was still there." At the grocery store, I shrugged off the bagger's offer to help me to the car. "No, thanks," I would reply. "This is the only exercise I get." I laughed, but the jokes were on me. They're on you too.

The Defiant Ones

Even mean-faced Defiant Woman, who pretends she's proud to have four chins and twice as many fat rolls, operates from shame. She may post Facebook photos of herself with a feast of artery-clogging food spread on the table. She could be eating a plateful of greasy ribs or a quart-size casserole dish full of macaroni and cheese. She might be dining on an elaborate meal or snapping a pic of her favorite dessert. Her expression is always the same: the bold stare right in the camera, forkful of food held high.

The Defiant Man isn't any different. He's the one who's had a heart attack or been diagnosed with Type 2 diabetes or already has had stents implanted to open his clogged arteries but continues to eat the foods that put him in the hospital in the first place. He's proud he's survived this long and doesn't intend to change now. He expects the medical profession to save him from himself. He's often outwardly angry. Nothing is good enough, everyone is out to get him or piss him off, and he's usually spoiling for a fight. Often, he has a tongue that could cut steel. He'll post pictures of his unhealthy plate piled high and add a comment that anyone who doesn't love what he loves is either lying or deranged.

The Defiant Ones may look you right in the eye while shoveling in the food and either act as if they don't care how big they are or as if they believe the big is beautiful lie, but their defensive anger comes from the humiliation of always being the fattest one in the room.

Permanent Victim

Permanent Victim believes she can't lose the flab no matter how hard she tries, so she might as well keep eating. She doesn't have time to exercise. She's stressed, unhappy, or angry. She's tired. She deserves whatever she's shoving in her face. This one may blame her family for not wanting to jump on the fitness wagon with her and complains that she cannot possibly cook one meal for them and another for herself.

One afternoon, I listened to a woman complain, while eating what must have been at least a 2,000-calorie chopped salad, that she could not lose the fat roll around her belly no matter how many sit-ups she did. I saw the bacon, avocado, chicken, and eggs mixed into a bowl of greens, all smothered with ranch dressing. All she saw was a salad. Just as I'd repeatedly done, she had tried a long list of weight-loss plans and products. Nothing worked because it was easier to tell herself she worked as hard as she could, but still didn't get the results she wanted. She kept gaining weight and finally developed Type 2 diabetes and high blood pressure.

I'm guilty of playing every one of these roles. Maybe you have too. I told my friends between bites of lava cake and ice cream that I deserved to splurge because of a rotten day at work. I rationalized the poison I fed my family. I quoted the food-is-my-only-pleasure line as a joke to friends.

Save the Excuses

No matter how I put them into words or how you may today, your excuses for staying fat are just that. Excuses. Family won't change their eating habits? Make the first change by cooking healthier meals. Can't ever lose no matter what you try? Start by driving by the drive-thru. I wish I had.

My worst shameful moment came two years after I joined *Cosmo*. I was preparing for our annual radio show, which we recorded in late December. One morning, my producer called and invited me to New York to tape the show. I would be able to meet all the people with whom I had become long-distance friends and visit the magazine's offices.

I should have been thrilled. Instead, my hands turned clammy and my heart pounded with anxiety. Although I desperately wanted to go, I could not bear to show up in the headquarters of the world's most glamorous women's magazine looking like I had flunked out of fat camp. So I lied. I told her I had a houseful of company coming for the holidays and that I just couldn't get away. No one was coming. Inner Bitch had beaten me into the ground. The mortifying shame of being fat and the horrifying fear that they would no longer like me or want me to work with them kept me home.

They never asked again. Even if they had, I wouldn't have gone because I was too ashamed of the way I looked. How many times have you passed up an opportunity you really wanted because of your size?

Try Shock Treatment

You know the sick, shocked feeling you get after you've caught a horrifying glimpse of your big butt in the bathroom mirror? Or when shopping, after you see your reflection in a storefront window and for an instant think, *Who is that fat woman?*

Those images are terrible, but rarely do they result in any serious change. In fact, they can produce an opposite effect, like rushing for a bag of Fritos and a tub of onion dip. At least that's what I did. Catching myself by surprise and seeing how I really looked usually sent me straight to the nearest Taco Bell.

Those random shocks of the brutal truth were too much to take. Well, maybe shock treatment was just what I needed.

As I learned that shame is the driving emotion behind most of our self-defeating actions, I began to wonder what would happen if we stuffed ourselves with shame. You know, like cigarette addicts who are forced to smoke until they vomit and can't stand to look at any form of tobacco again.

The fatter I became, the more I avoided looking at anything but my face in the mirror. Sound familiar? Then try this. Stand naked in front of your mirror and take a hard, long look at yourself. Inspect every pucker, crease, and fold. Then think about the loaded potato or meatball sandwich or quart of ice cream you're about to eat. I know you want it. However, your swollen, unhealthy body is the proof that not only could you live for a couple of months on nothing but water and lettuce, but that you're slowly killing yourself.

If you do this experiment, know that Inner Bitch will try anything to get you to eat the crap you're craving. She may squeal like the pig she is and tell you you're hopeless so eat up. She may try the best-friend routine and say that you don't really look that bad. Whatever you hear in your head that doesn't tell you to throw the garbage you've been eating into the trash and reach for a healthy alternative is her lying voice. The thought of seeing your bare-assed, overstuffed, overworked, and chemically poisoned body might just kill your appetite.

I'll make you another bet. Even if you never really eat naked in front of a mirror, now that you have the image in your head, maybe that vision will help you take one less mouthful of poison and one more step back to health. I hope so.

CHAPTER 5

IT'S ONLY ONE DAY

How many times have you decided to get healthy right after the holidays? Every January 1, losing weight and exercising are the top New Year's resolutions. But, even before Super Bowl Sunday, 80 percent of those vows are forgotten.[1]

After the holiday feeding frenzy, once again, I made my inevitable pledge to go on another diet. Inner Bitch didn't say a word. She didn't have to. For two weeks, I starved and managed to lose five pounds. Then, just as I began to feel human again, Super Bowl Sunday roared into the driveway, tailgate flapping, loaded with hot wings, stuffed jalapeños, and supermarket meat-and-cheese platters. The bowl of ranch dip sitting in the middle of a token vegetable plate negated any health benefits of that snack. Did I care? No. It was only one day.

Just one day to celebrate. But just as you wipe the last smear of wing sauce off your face, you turn around and, oops, it's Valentine's Day. Break out the candy hearts and, if you are romantic, a cozy champagne-drenched dinner for two. Or post Instagram photos of yourself sitting behind an oversize dessert, justifying your behavior because that special day only happens once a year. But by the time you've finished flossing the chocolate-covered almonds out of your teeth, St. Patrick swings by. Even if you're not a fan of corned beef, cabbage, and green beer, there are plenty of other options to help celebrate this festive day. Shamrock-shaped sugar cookies. Irish coffee. Chocolate "gold" coins.

You don't get a chance to catch your breath before the Easter bunny hops in, dragging a basketful of chocolate bunnies behind him. Add a ham dinner to rival Thanksgiving and assorted cream pies for dessert. Who could pass up this celebration? Not I. Then, before the dye dries on the eggs, Mother's Day rings the doorbell. Chances are, if we are overweight, so is Mom. So what do we do? Take her out for a calorie-loaded dinner that is sure to raise both her cholesterol and her blood pressure. Ours too. No worries. It's only one day.

How many times have you done the same thing? Whether it is Super Bowl Sunday or a personal celebration, once special-occasion amnesia kicks in, we develop tunnel vision and conveniently forget how often these events happen. They rise like the tide, and we wade in with any lame excuse that gives us a reason to eat.

Soon, school is out, and Memorial Day weekend rolls around to kick-start summer with the first official barbecue of the season. Ribs, chicken, a side of cow, all smothered in sauce. Potato salad. Hot dogs. Beans and bacon. Anything and bacon.

Father's Day is next on the menu. All Dad wants to do is flop in front of the sports channel and eat, and we are happy to accommodate him. Spread out the food on the coffee table, wrap a beach towel around his neck, and he could chomp himself into a heart attack. Before you hand him that extra serving of ribs while he's sitting on the couch, think about what you're really serving. Yes, it's only one day, but he has only one life.

During the first half of the year, I managed to lose—and then gain back—fifteen pounds, give or take a pound. *Cosmo* asked me to write a daily horoscope for its new website. My second book was almost finished, and I still worked full time. The opportunities were amazing. The stress drove my personal food fiend insane. A friend asked me how I could have consciously thought I could eat like that and not gain weight. Was she kidding? I didn't think. No overweight person consciously thinks about what they are eating while they are eating. Only after they are sick from a food overdose do they consider the damage. Even then, the odds are, as soon as the nausea subsides, they reach for more food. On the rare occasions I forced myself to face the facts, I felt guilty and ashamed. Still, I didn't accept responsibility for my behavior. Nor did I seriously consider what I was doing to my health. Instead, I told myself that I knew what I was doing and could control myself. Of course, I didn't.

Summer arrived with a bang on the Fourth of July, another grillin'-and-chillin' holiday. Although our local minor-league baseball team hosts a fireworks display after their annual holiday game, I don't like to sit in a grandstand in one-hundred-plus degree heat and have my eardrums shattered. Hauling an over two-hundred-pound body up the steps is grueling, and it's nearly impossible to walk down, and then lumber back up while carrying a plate of food, and a twenty-ounce cup of Coke. So I stayed home and watched the pyrotechnics from the comfort of the couch while eating homemade chicken nachos.

July through August is vacation time, and who counts calories at the beach or in the mountains or at Disneyland? Not I. The whole point of vacation is to avoid cooking, right? Besides, we always do enough walking to negate anything we eat. So we think. These are the days we take the kids to the nearest amusement park, camp out, head for the in-laws in another state, or visit a national park. Whatever happens, obese people cannot diet on vacation. We tell ourselves that is the only time we can truly relax, so we gladly and guiltlessly live on artificially flavored, microwaved, over-processed, and nitrate-filled nonfood.

As soon we are home and the car is unpacked, Labor Day weekend and the last binge of the season arrive. Then the kids head back to school, and you and I head, credit card in hand, to the nearest diet center. That lasts about four weeks, until Halloween creeps in, clutching three-pound bags of candy, which I always cherry-pick before handing out to the trick-or-treaters.

Guess what? You, me, and every other overweight person in the country has come full circle and are packing our bags for the next trip into the Bermuda Triangle of holiday food benders.

Add to this list Hanukkah, Eid-ul-fitr, Kwanzaa, and a multitude of other religious or spiritual festivities. Between the holidays, squeeze in weddings, showers, anniversaries, birthdays, funerals, Sunday dinners, and other personal celebrations. Add the casual lunches and dinners out with friends. Overweight people have a built-in tunnel vision that only focuses on the next event, which absolves us from thinking we are in a never-ending cycle. The annual holiday binge is only the beginning. There will always be one more party or I-deserve-this day. Our over-stuffed brains never manage to add up the number of celebrations because we're stuck in the denial of *it's only one day*.

Out of a fifty-two-week year, most people resolve to lose weight the week after New Year's and the week after Labor Day. Think about it. Two weeks out of an entire year, we attempt to try again.

Instead of making food the focal point of any party or my life, I have learned to listen to my body. I eat when it's hungry, not when my head is. I lost 122 pounds in three years. But my journey as an unhealthy, overweight woman in denial took more than twenty. Yours can be much shorter. You know that within the next month, perhaps week, you will celebrate something. Celebrate the person, or holiday, not the food. You can do it. Then when your birthday rolls around again, you'll be able to celebrate yourself and give yourself the best gift of all. Your health.

CHAPTER 6

LOSING FOR ALL THE WRONG REASONS

Your class reunion is in three months. You've packed on the pounds since college, and you starve yourself for weeks so you can brag that you're still the size you were at twenty. A friend asks you to be in her wedding. You sign up for a commercial weight-loss program because you cannot imagine squeezing into a bridesmaid's dress at your current size. Whatever the reason, you rush for the latest fad or fall back on a previous program that worked before in hopes that you can dump ten or twenty or thirty pounds as quickly as possible. Losing for any goal other than your own long-term health automatically sets you up for failure.

The Big Event

You might panic if you've been asked to be a bridesmaid, but what if you are the bride? Sixty percent of brides-to-be go on some kind of diet before their wedding, and some of the draconian efforts they use might explain why so many turn into bridezillas. They may use diet pills or skip meals or go to extremes, as with the HCG diet.[1]

HCG (human chorionic gonadotropin) is a naturally-occurring pregnancy hormone. As a prescription medication, it's used to treat fertility issues in women. The HCG diet consists of taking pills or liquids containing this substance that are usually labeled "homeopathic," one of those words that lead consumers to believe this stuff is safe. It isn't. The FDA warns of possible links to cancer. The weight quickly falls off, but the real reason it does is because the diet restricts calories to just 500 to 800 per day. Maybe that's why some brides faint at the altar. And don't let your guy anywhere near this mess, either. A bridegroom taking it could end up with boobs bigger than yours.

One woman I knew was determined to lose seventy-five pounds before her big day. She used SlimFast shakes and bars supplemented with a daily salad. Although she lost most of the weight and looked wonderful on her wedding day, within a few months, she had regained almost every pound.

I know that feeling well. Whenever I wanted to drop a fast five or ten pounds, SlimFast was my grocery-store go-to plan because it was so easy. Two meal replacements, chosen from a variety of bars and shakes, one 500-calorie meal, and three of their 100-calorie snacks during the day. The pre-made shakes were my favorite, and I couldn't tell you how many gallons I drank over the course of my battle with my weight. The advertisements tell us these concoctions are rich in protein and vitamins, which we assume means healthy. You decide. The first three ingredients of the shakes are water, milk protein concentrate, and canola oil, followed by a list of sugars, artificial flavors, and preservatives.[2] No wonder one of the side effects is diarrhea.

The SlimFast Keto diet plan includes Fat Bomb meal bars and snacks. One of the main ingredients listed is an MCT (medium-chain triglyceride) blend of palm and coconut oils and grass-fed butter—pure saturated fat. One Fat Bomb meal contains twelve grams of this heart-clogging mixture.[3]

Not long after S. Daniel Abraham came home from World War II and went to work in his uncle's drug company in New York, he decided he could do better. Seeing an advertisement for itch-relief cream, Abraham talked to the small manufacturer and ended up buying both the product and the business for five thousand dollars. Then he packed his suitcase and became a traveling salesman. Abraham traveled through several neighboring states, where he handed out samples of his new product to doctors and pharmacists and tacked up advertising posters in every town. Soon, business was booming, and the kid formed the Thompson Medical Company. He hired chemists and pharmacologists to tweak products manufactured by other companies and continued to buy more small companies.

In 1956, Abraham jumped into the diet industry. His first product, Slim-Mint gum, a concoction full of the appetite suppressant and tongue-numbing benzocaine, was a wild success. Next, he added Figure-Aid, one of the amphetamine-laden diet pills that were all the rage during the sixties. In 1976, he hit the big time with Dexatrim. This pill was full of PPA (phenylpropanolamine), commonly used as a prescription to treat nasal congestion and allergies. A side effect was loss of appetite due to frequent nausea and the fact that users lost their senses of taste and smell. Food just didn't appear appetizing in any way. How convenient. So, of course, this toxin was dumped into other diet products flooding the market at the time. That is, until young women between the ages of eighteen and twenty-one starting dying from hemorrhagic strokes, and the FDA stopped the sales of PPA-laced products. No worries for Abraham though. Thanks to Dexatrim, he'd already raked in $50 million.

Ever the cutting-edge entrepreneur, his labs next engineered SlimFast powder. After a setback in 1977, the boy genius went public, and the stock offering netted him $8.4 million, which saved the company and enabled him to hit the SlimFast marketing hard.

At the same time, Thompson Medical was churning out Aspercream, Sportscreme, and Cortozone-5, but by 1990, SlimFast was earning so much money that Abraham spun off a company just for the diet products. In 2000, he sold SlimFast to Unilever for a staggering $2.4 billion. Since then, the company has changed hands a few more times, most recently selling to global group Glanbia for a paltry $350 million, reflecting an overall declining interest in over-the-counter diet products. Although this downward trend is directly connected to more people opting to eat healthier, for every product that disappears or sells fewer items, a dozen more pop up like weeds in the grocery aisles.[4]

Before taking an anniversary cruise, a friend of mine went on the Hollywood 48-Hour Miracle Diet, followed by another two weeks of near-starvation, to lose more than twenty pounds.

No one knows exactly who invented this one, but rumor has it that a famous movie star of the forties commissioned one of the Mayo brothers to develop the juice. Although probably untrue, the glamour of Hollywood and the prestige of Dr. Mayo sent this product to the head of the line for quick weight reduction. Still popular today, the ads promise extreme results. One headline screams, "Lose up to 10 Pounds in 48 Hours!" I can see why. Basically, this is a blend of fruit juice concentrates, vitamins, and essential oils. For two days, you drink a mixture of four ounces of juice and four ounces of water four times a day. You drink an additional eight glasses of water each day. At 100 calories per serving, you're consuming 400 calories a day. You're not allowed any other food or beverages, including alcohol, caffeine, or tobacco. You will lose quickly, in part because of the effects of that much concentrated fruit juice, and because you'll be peeing every thirty minutes. You won't lose fat. You may suffer from hypoglycemia (low blood sugar), which can cause shakiness, headaches, weakness, anxiety, and confusion. Even this plan warns you not to use the juice more often than once a week and advises customers to "maintain a sensible eating plan and exercise regularly."[5]

My friend lost the weight, made herself sick in the process, and spent the first two days of the voyage in their cabin. Once she felt well enough to eat again, she took advantage of the endless buffet aboard ship. By the time the trip ended ten days later, she'd gained back eight pounds.

Forget these drastic promises of the diet industry. Nothing works permanently except consistent, committed effort.

The Person You Want to Impress

A woman I knew had struggled with her weight for most of her adult life. As I had, she cycled through one program after another, trying to find some way to keep the weight off. Nothing worked for long. When romance entered her life, she resorted to lap band surgery because she wanted to lose as much weight as she could in the shortest possible time. Within a couple of months, she lost forty pounds. Then another thirty or so melted away. The affair ended as quickly as it had flared. She changed jobs, moved to another city, and gained back every ounce.

My worst diet failure happened when I finally agreed to meet my *Cosmo* editor and had six months to lose fifty pounds. I panicked and waddled straight to the then-newest fad, LA Weight Loss.

43

The center looked like a doctor's office with a small reception area and chairs sitting against the walls. I signed in, sat down, and watched a looping video showing before-and-after photos of smiling men and women testifying on behalf of the program. The only reading materials were the usual propaganda fliers and their cookbook for sale at $19.95.

After a short wait, a counselor took me into a private office and began the sales pitch. No meetings. No appointments. I could weigh in every day if I wanted. They offered five plans in descending order of calories I could eat and increasing in the length of time of the program. All included LA Lite snack bars in a variety of flavors and chocolate or vanilla protein shake mixes.

The plans were nothing more than portion-controlled, low-calorie, high-protein diets, which produced a slow, steady loss. At $250 for twenty weeks, the plan itself was relatively inexpensive. That price included private weigh-ins and talks with the counselor, a.k.a. salesperson. They made their money on the snack bars you were required to buy, the shake mixes, and a variety of vitamins and mineral supplements they pushed. I walked out of the center with a shopping bag full of nonfood and an invoice in my purse for $1400.

I lost forty-seven pounds, looked and felt great, and was eager to meet the editor with whom I'd become long-distance friends. Then he called to tell me that he had pneumonia and had to cancel his trip. At that moment, I emotionally canceled my diet.

I limped along on the plan for a few more weeks, but soon, and in her friendliest voice, Inner Bitch began to come up with all kinds of excuses to eat. *Reward yourself every time you lose five more pounds. Just have one piece of candy or one cookie. Eat what you want in moderation. Cheat one day and jump right back on track the next. Eat. Eat. Eat.*

Of course, no matter what I ate, I still had the LA Lites energy bars. The snack bars provided extra protein to curb my appetite between meals. One bar also provided eighteen grams (72 percent) of the American Heart Association's recommended daily amount of twenty-six grams of sugar. In fact, I got hooked on the candy bar taste and would eat up to four of the 170-calorie snacks a day. I would have been better off if I'd just eaten a couple of Snickers.[6]

I justified my latest disaster by telling myself that at least I wouldn't gain back what it had cost me a house payment to lose. Wrong. By the time I did meet my editor, I'd regained thirty-five pounds, and all I could think was how fat and ugly I must look to someone who looked like a model himself. I failed because I didn't lose weight to become healthy. I lost to impress him. That episode began another downward spiral of overeating in which I regained the whole forty-seven pounds I'd lost plus eighty-five more.

Even if my editor hadn't canceled his first trip, my outcome would have been the same. No woman on the planet wants to be the biggest one in the room. However, losing weight just to look good for someone else might as well come with a guarantee that you'll gain back every ounce.

The fear of being embarrassed, or falling in love, or seeking revenge will never lead to permanent weight loss. These temporary fixes fail every time because the only motivation for permanent weight loss should be to save your health and your life.

The Perfect Body

The word diet comes from the Greek *diaita*, which represented a way of life that included food, drink, lifestyle, and exercise. With the exceptions of running naked in public and regular vomiting, the Greeks' basic idea was close to our idea of healthy today. Where the concept gets skewed is in body image. In ancient Greece, the ideal body was male, slim, muscular, and handsome—the Greek god image. The ideal woman was rounder, with full hips and breasts, which represented fertility and motherhood. This concept changed over the centuries until in the Victorian age when the vision of an ideal woman included a tiny waist and slender body. Women aimed for an hourglass figure by cinching their waists with corsets and girdles so tight they couldn't eat, could barely breathe, and often fainted. Men wore them too, to pull in their middle-aged paunches.

In the 1920s, rubberized versions of corsets and girdles were sold as a quick way to sweat off the fat. The gimmick was that you would lose fat and look slimmer at the same time. In reality, all these irritating rigs did was cause heat rash. The water you lost from sweating was minimal and temporary. That didn't stop this fad from recycling through the mid-2000s when the celebrity body wrap became all the rage. This version didn't stop at just a corset. Your whole body was wrapped tighter than Cleopatra's mummy, and then you sweated your guts out for about ninety minutes, as you supposedly lost a dress size or two. Hollywood A-listers suffered this treatment to look hot on the red carpet. Soon, even your hometown spa offered some sort of body wrap to squeeze off the pounds. You had to keep up the expensive treatments, because as soon as you unwrapped and had a glass of water, your body began to replenish the moisture that had just been wrung out of it.

A friend of mine subjected herself to a body wrap in order to fit into a bridesmaid's dress that was a little too tight for her comfort. She had her waist and hips bound tightly for about ninety minutes while she lay on a table at a health spa. She looked great at the wedding. The dress fit perfectly and her figure had a definite hourglass shape. The effects lasted for a couple of days, and then her figure returned to its pre-wrap size.

Another friend tried the whole-body wrap. This one was an herbal wrap infused with herbs and scents that were supposed to help relax and detox her while she was being temporarily mummified. Although she was already tiny, the wrap did take a couple of pounds of water out of her system, but the aftereffects were the same.

The wraps are still around, and many of the places that use them today are owned by doctors. The medical spa offers everything from body wraps to diet plans to Botox, all under the supervision of a doctor. These are even more expensive because of their connection to a physician. However, none of the results are permanent. You have to keep getting wrapped, injected, sliced, lasered, or starved to maintain the look you desire. I'm all for having the best body and skin possible, but you can have it without either the excessive cost or wild treatments of some of these places.

A plant-based diet naturally clears your body of harmful toxins that help both your skin and your figure. Most important, moving to a diet of plant-based foods helps your body heal itself from the inside instead of just making you temporarily look better on the outside.

CHAPTER 7

FALLING FOR EVERY FAD

How many times have you fallen for an old scam or new fad that promises you will lose ten pounds or more in two weeks? In my hundreds of attempts to lose weight, I've tried more diets than I care to count. I've bought dozens of exercise gadgets too.

Whether it's an established program endorsed by a celebrity, the diet center down the street, or the latest wonder pill, these modern snake oil peddlers are experts in knowing how to get and keep your business by promising the most results for the least effort.

Every day, we are bombarded with fast-food commercials for meals that load us with fat and salt and cholesterol, followed by commercials for programs guaranteed to help us shed those ugly extra pounds. These are followed by more commercials for hundreds of different kinds of pills, drinks, and powders, each one promising to make us lose weight without much work on our part. All we have to do is believe the hype and hand over our cash. What do these rip-offs have in common? Each has side effects ranging from oily diarrhea to heart failure, and the one constant in this insanity is that they all come with a recommended low-fat, low-calorie diet plan. Yet, despite the money we pour down this endless black hole, obesity rates in every developed country around the world are climbing, with the United States ranked twelfth of 191 nations.

Bizarre weight-loss methods have been around for centuries and show to what lengths people will go to slim down—not to be confused with getting healthy—and how easily big marketing campaigns can sucker us into believing they have a simple fix for our unending fight against obesity.

Have a Smoke

In 1928, the American Tobacco Company told its consumers that smoking was not only good for them, but that puffing a pack of cigarettes could help them lose weight. Lucky Strike was one brand that seized on this deadly idea and ran a series of magazine advertisements. One full-page ad assured potential buyers cigarettes were safe because "20,679 physicians put themselves on record in confirming the fact that toasting makes Lucky Strikes less irritating to the throat than any other brand." The claim was that toasting the tobacco "removes impurities" and "makes them a delightful alternative for things that make you fat."[1]

At the time, the medical profession had no idea of the link between smoking and lung cancer. Only in the 1940s, after a lung cancer epidemic swept the globe, did medical science begin to make a connection between the two. Twenty years later, even as doctors died right along with their patients, the medical profession was still making up its collective mind about the dangers of smoking. That delay helped the cigarette and funeral industries gain more customers.

Another ad, "Reach for a Lucky Instead," specifically aimed at women, promised them this was an easy way to remain slim. For the times, the campaign was considered a bold move because the idea of women smoking in public was not widely accepted. Although it appeared as a cutting-edge endorsement of the then-modern woman, it perpetuated the idea that women should lose weight just to be appealing to men. The health consequences were never a factor.[2]

Eat All You Want—of Just One Food

Recycled for the twenty-first century, the dangerous and boring mono diet consists of eating just one food for a couple of weeks as a fast way to lose weight. The food you choose doesn't matter. You could eat bananas or carrots or even chocolate, but that's all you eat for at least fourteen consecutive days.

Who would do such a ridiculous thing? Plenty of people, including celebrity magician Penn Jillette. Instead of astounding one of his Las Vegas audiences by making an elephant disappear, Jillette amazed the country by losing 104 pounds in four months. Definitely don't try this trick at home.[3]

At 322 pounds and dangerously ill, Jillette called his friend, Ray Cronise, a former NASA engineer-turned-weight-loss-coach. Although Cronise has alluded to creating the potato version of the mono diet, this fad has been around since 1849. The original plan promised overweight men that they would become lean and required them to stay on the potatoes-only menu for three to five days once a month. More than 160 years later, the potato diet is still hyped as another fast cure for obesity.

Jillette ate nothing but potatoes for two weeks. Nothing. He could eat russets, fingerlings, Yukon Gold, or any other type he craved. He could boil them, bake them, or eat them raw. He had to eat them plain—no salt, oil, or sour cream—and was allowed up to five per day. Then gradually, more vegetables, fruits, and whole grains were added until he was eating about 1,200 calories per day.[4]

You would think that, after such an extreme weight loss, Penn Jillette would be the first to promote this plan to anyone within earshot. Not so. Instead, he told Dr. Oz, *USA Today*, and a slew of others that this diet is not for everyone. He's adamant about it. A lineup of physicians, nutritionists, and weight-loss experts agree with him. At an average intake of 800 calories per day and no balanced nutrition, this fad can result in anything from dizziness to a trip to the hospital.

Plus, while quickly losing a huge amount of weight looks dramatic, and it is tempting to think that you could be five or six sizes smaller within a few months, rapid weight loss sets the stage for gallstones and fatty liver disease. You could lose more water and lean muscle tissue than actual fat. If you're still tempted to try this diet, though, Jillette has some words for you: "If you're getting medical advice from a Las Vegas magician, you are making bad life choices."[5]

Satisfy Your Sweet Tooth

Have a cookie. Chocolate is great. Caramel is fabulous. Cinnabon tastes just like that drool-worthy bun you can buy at the fair. Would you rather have candy? Or a granola bar? No problem. When all else fails, you can buy a product that supposedly tricks your mind into thinking you're eating a snack instead of a diet aid. What you're really getting is fleeced by clever marketing ploys designed to separate you from your money in any possible way.

When it hit the market in the 1930s, Ayds Reducing Plan Candy was an instant success. At two dollars for a thirty-day supply, it was cheap even then. The idea was simple. Eat two reducing candies with hot tea or coffee before each meal as an appetite suppressant. You didn't even have to follow a specific plan because you would automatically eat less by taking Ayds.[6]

Until 1945, the company raked in the profits. Then, an advertisement stating, "100 Fat Ladies Lose 20lbs. Each," caught the attention of the Federal Trade Commission. The ad claimed that these women took part in a thirty-day clinical study and that all of them lost at least twenty pounds. Not true. The FTC told the manufacturer to rein it in, and the company pulled the ad. Then, the FTC went further and had the ingredients analyzed to ensure the diet candy didn't contain any of the several drug compounds used in other diet products. Ayds passed the drug test. But the test revealed the real secret to the product's enormous popularity. It *was* candy. Plain caramel candy in a variety of flavors with some vitamins tossed in so it could pretend to be a diet aid. The government pulled the plug on the phony advertising, and for a couple of years, the company eased up on its wilder statements. Then a revamped formula hit the market. The new Ayds included benzocaine, the main ingredient in Orajel. The idea was to desensitize your tongue so food didn't taste as good. The ads stopped talking about fat women losing weight and shifted to celebrity endorsements from some of Hollywood's A-list stars of the day. At the time, Campana, a division of Purex, owned Ayds, and its president, Irving Crull, maintained the celebrity tie-ins by having friends like Hedy Lamarr and other movie stars churn out new advertisements. This kept the candy a hot-selling item until the 1970s, when the ads started looking like headlines from the *National Enquirer*. One read, "I Got Stuck in a Church Pew Before I Lost 70 Pounds." Believe it or not, this switch resulted in even bigger sales, and Ayds remained one of the best weight-loss scams on the market. Then everything came crashing down. In 1981, Purex sold the brand to Jeffrey

Martin, Inc. Not long after, the AIDS epidemic struck. The new owners were advised to rename the product if they wanted the diet candy to survive. They refused, arguing that forty years of success would shield the product against the fallout from the unfortunately similar name. It didn't. Consumers shunned the product, and it disappeared from the market, as it should have decades before.[7]

Fueled by our attraction to anything that remotely resembles dessert or a forbidden treat, cookies and candies that are supposed to help us lose weight are still popular today. They all work the same way. Either eat them before meals to help control your appetite, or as a meal replacement. Cookies for breakfast? Irresistible.

Since 1975, Dr. Siegel's Cookie Diet has been advertised as eating "normal" cookies that contain a "special mixture of proteins that naturally suppress hunger." They also contain mostly salt and sugar. You eat nine of the sixty-calorie cookies a day and either a 500 or 700 calorie dinner depending on how fast you want to lose. The idea of eating cookies all day may seem ideal, but the plan doesn't teach you anything about maintaining healthy eating habits or making lifestyle changes, so when you stop the cookies, the weight returns. This one comes with a costly recommendation not to try it without a doctor's supervision. Could that be because this diet doesn't supply enough nutrients to sustain your body long term?[8]

The Hollywood Cookie Diet (cousin to the Hollywood Miracle Juice you just read about) advertises that each cookie is a healthy meal substitute. You eat four cookies a day—breakfast, mid-morning snack, lunch, and afternoon snack—followed by what the ad calls a "sensible dinner." The instructions advise you to "exercise regularly, it's good for your heart and good for your figure." Regular exercise is very good for your heart. These 150-calorie-each cookies aren't. The first five ingredients in the chocolate chip flavor are flour, chocolate chips (sugar, cocoa butter, and soy lecithin), cane syrup, cane sugar, and palm oil. You may be eating only 600 calories, but the majority of those are processed sugar.[9]

Love gummy candies? This mix of sugar, gelatin, and various flavors comes in all sorts of shapes and sizes.

Unless you buy gelatin products made with agar-agar, a seaweed extract, your favorite chewy snack or jiggly Jell-O contains basically what's swept off the slaughterhouse floor. Hides and bones from animals killed for food.[10]

If that doesn't bother you, you can buy diet gummies too. SkinnyMint sells "super fat-burning gummies," that come in two flavors. Power Up is apple-flavored and contains 400 milligrams of green coffee bean extract. The instructions say to take two with breakfast for a boost of energy to start the day. Hunger Buster gummies are strawberry-flavored appetite suppressants that contain 500 milligrams of garcinia cambogia extract. The company also sells Morning Boost and Night Cleanse teas. You get more caffeine with the morning tea and a dose of senna, a natural laxative, at night. Basically, what you're taking is a mixture that does little more than give you the jitters and diarrhea. Although none of the ingredients are especially harmful, garcinia cambogia can have negative interactions with several medications, such as allergy and asthma meds, blood thinners, cholesterol-lowering drugs, pain and anxiety medications, and others. The website advises that these products should be used, "with a reduced-calorie diet and regular exercise program for maximum results." Nothing new here.[11]

Fill Up on Cabbage Soup

This is another fad that rears its ugly head every few years. I tried it a few times and can tell you it's not for the fainthearted. But at one time it was so popular that even *Cosmopolitan* published an article about its benefits.[12]

The soup consists of a head of chopped cabbage, onions, boxed onion soup mix, bell peppers, celery, vegetable juice, water, and spices. You eat as much of this as you can stand and add various combinations of fruits and vegetables as the week wears on. Believe me; it wears on and on and on. One day, you eat soup and bananas. The next day, it might be soup and any fruit but bananas. The plan boasts that you will lose up to ten pounds in seven days. I tried this one a couple of times and lost between six and seven pounds each time. But I could not stand the regimen for more than a week. Sure, it works, but like every other drastic plan, as soon as you stop, the weight piles back on.

Eat Your Favorite Fast Food

When the low-fat craze became as popular as dropping by a drive-thru on the way home from work, the fast-food chains were eager to grab as much of the market as they could.

In 1991, McDonalds introduced the McLean Deluxe burger. To cut the fat to ten grams, from the twenty-six grams in a Big Mac, the company added water and seaweed to the beef. The sodium levels were high at 670 grams, and they still slapped on a slice of that plastic-like processed cheese that never quite melts. The only lean thing about this short-lived sandwich was its name.[13]

Today, vegan meat substitutes have become fixtures on the menus of fast-food chains like Carl's Jr., White Castle, Burger King, and KFC. You can get tacos, burgers, and meatless chicken nuggets along with your fries, sodas, and a variety of toppings. Don't be fooled. Just because it's vegan doesn't necessarily mean it's healthy or calorie-friendly. Many of these products are heavily processed. When you load your meatless burger with cheese, special sauce, onion rings—or any combination of those—and then pack it into a processed bun, about the only nutritional gain is the absence of actual beef and its high saturated-fat content.

Making your own meatless favorites is easier than you think. I've included some easy dishes in the recipe section.

Just as with processed foods, you shouldn't automatically believe a label that says vegan or vegetarian or plant-based is healthy.

Take More Pills

If you aren't being sold fat disguised as healthy food, you're being sold placebos sold as magic pills that make calories disappear.

Alli, popular and cheap at $4.99 per bottle, says it can help you lose "a significant amount of belly fat in about twelve weeks." If you haven't tried this little wonder yet, you should know that much of the extra weight you lose is the result of the horrendous case of greasy diarrhea it gives you. The main ingredient, orlistat, is a fat-binding drug prescribed in larger doses by doctors. Alli contains 60 mg of orlistat. Its prescription big brother, Xenical, contains 120mg. From the stories I've heard from people who have taken Alli and had to practically live in the bathroom, I cannot imagine what Xenical would do to someone's body. Once you've had enough belly aches and decide to drop the bottle in the trash, the weight comes right back. Yes, it also comes with the standard recommendation to eat a healthy diet and keep up the exercise.[14]

The fads and diets I've described are only a small fraction of plans on the market today. They may seem easy. They promise results. But, I believe, the only real value in any of these over-the-counter products is the advice some of them offer to eat a well-balanced diet low in fats and sugar. Eating cookies may be fun, and quick-loss juices may help you to drop a few pounds in a short time, but these products, and others like them, don't teach you how to permanently keep the weight off.

Shake, Rattle, and Roll

Assuming that you lived through the various crazy diets, but were still stuck at a depressing weight, there was and still is a whole other world of gimmicks guaranteed to make you look like a super-star in no time.

Vibrating your fat off became popular in the 1930s and recycles through the fitness world about every twenty years. The original machine was a heavy-duty platform you stood on, and then you strapped a wide belt around your butt or your thighs or whatever part of your body wanted to slim, flipped a switch, and held on tight. Invented in the late 1800s, one shook you until your teeth rattled. These and other types of "passive exercise" equipment were designed so you didn't have to do any work. All you did was stand, sit, or lie down while the machines rolled, twisted, or vibrated the fat off your flabby body.

In the 1970s and '80s, the Gloria Marshall Figure Salons revived these methods. The bait was a series of commercials showing women wearing cute sweaters, shorts, and heels while moving from one machine to the next. Another showed over-weight women not even breathing hard while strapped to the vibrating belt or sitting with an arm flung over a huge set of wooden rollers that pummeled their underarm flab. I tried this too. Of course, my reasoning was little effort for lots of gain. The only thing I gained was more pounds from the snacks I treated myself to after each session.[15]

Today, a whole new series of vibrating platforms promise to transform your body into one tight mass of sculpted muscle, all within the privacy of your home. They supposedly force your muscles to contract without you having to do anything. You can spend thousands of dollars on a professional machine, but most seem to fall in the two-hundred- to five-hundred-dollar range. You can even get an As-Seen-On-TV bargain platform for just $14.99 plus shipping. All come with some kind of advice to eat a balanced diet and add other exercises to your routine.[16]

Today, the medical profession is assessing the benefits of vibrating platforms, although the jury is still out on whether or not they truly are as beneficial as their advertisements claim. Advice from the Mayo Clinic suggests that whole-body vibration "may help with weight loss when you also cut back on calories." Further, the machines have not been shown to provide the same health benefits as walking, biking, or swimming. So why not save your money and get out in the fresh air and walk, bike, or swim?[17]

By the 1970s, people were wearing inflatable sauna pants to mold their bodies into shape. One brand, Wonder Sauna Hot Pants advertised that you would "look better, feel better, and wake up your body." These puffy shorts promised to sweat off the fat around your belly and thighs. Of course, they didn't work, but that didn't stop men and women from wasting money on them. Sauna belts were popular at the gym. You zipped this tight, rubberized belt around your waist, and then did your exercise program. You lost weight from sweating, but as soon as you took the thing off and had a drink of water, it came right back.[18]

Despite the fact that sauna belts did nothing to help with permanent weight loss or to reduce the size of your waist for other than a very short time, they are still popular today. You can get a waist trainer, body suit, sauna belt, or all kinds of stretchy fabrics that can be wound around any part of your body. All will wring you out for a few hours or overnight. None will help you make any permanent change.

From the Thigh Master to the Ab Roller to an all-in-one home gym, the list of exercise equipment is endless. All promise dramatic results with minimal effort. Most end up in the garage, the trash, or as a donation to your favorite charitable organization.

Do yourself a favor. Follow a healthy diet full of vegetables, grains, beans, and fruit. Stop eating highly processed foods, junk food, and fast food. Exercise in moderation. Forget these scams and just start moving forward. One choice. One bite. One day at a time.

Love Your Fat Body Just the Way It Is

The absolute worst scam isn't the next deadly diet. It's giving up on yourself and acting as if being overweight is just who you are or falling for the lie that being obese is okay.

Big is not beautiful. Fat is a living organism that will kill you. Beneath that pretty face your body is rotting, and no amount of glamour makeup or designer clothes can change that fact. Today, 300,000 people a year die prematurely from obesity-related diseases. Heart disease, diabetes, osteoporosis, and thirteen cancers have been linked to being overweight, and yet we just keep getting fatter.[19]

During the 2020 pandemic, a scary figure emerged as the disease spread. Obese people with COVID-19 were twice as likely to be admitted to the hospital and seven times more likely to need to be placed on a ventilator. Younger adults who were obese had similar risks, even though they might not have had any underlying health conditions.[20]

Overweight and obese men aren't immune from thinking that being fat is okay. When the term "dad bod" hit social media, the internet flipped. Dad bods are supposedly balanced somewhere between six-pack abs and a beer gut. The guy who owns one hits the gym on occasion and can put away eight slices of pizza in one sitting.

My head began to swim with images of Mr. Pepperoni Breath's sauce-splattered belly hanging over his flannel pajama bottoms. Maybe this is a joke, I thought. No such luck. Instead, the dad bod became one in a long line of unhealthy crazes sweeping our already overweight, out-of-shape country. Belly fat isn't limited to the paunch pushing against his shirt. It's surrounding and squeezing his internal organs. That extra bulge doubles his risk of heart disease and early death.

Remember that the next time you're rounding up the wings, chips and dips, or barbecue for his birthday or your next party like Super Bowl Sunday. That's the day the average American shovels in more than 2500 calories and 121 grams of fat during the four-hour chunk of time spent in front of the TV, screaming for their favorite team. It's no wonder that guy you care about is in a stupor after the game—that is, if he's not in an ambulance racing for the hospital.[21]

Regardless of what you hear or see on popular television shows, or read about online or in a magazine, an obese body is like a ticking bomb. Obesity is like the hub of a wheel with spokes that connect to every chronic condition and major disease you can suffer. It's not glamorous. It's deadly.

CHAPTER 8

WEIGHT WATCHERS, NUTRISYSTEM & JENNY CRAIG: THE BEASTS THAT WILL NOT DIE

Would you go to a doctor with a patient death rate of 95 percent? Neither would I. Yet, Weight Watchers, Nutrisystem, and Jenny Craig want you to believe that their long-term failure rates of an average 95 percent are successful.[1]

These three companies alone rake in almost $3 billion annually by hooking us with promises of amazing results.[2]

From a business viewpoint, it's a genius move because customers think they're being coached and supported, but all they get are emotional strokes from trained salespeople. They empty our wallets while knowing that we will fail, and keep failing, until their bank accounts are fatter than our spreading asses. What we spend is astronomically high, but the emotional cost of repeated failure is even higher.

The come-ons are similar—eat the foods you love and still lose weight. However, what you are really doing is eating fewer calories of the same unhealthy food you ate before. If that isn't enough, each of these corporations pushes its own line of fat-, carb-, and sugar-loaded frozen products.

All hire celebrities to hawk their programs and products, but if you look at those celebrities' failures, you'll see that the rich and famous don't seem to have any better results at permanent weight loss than their members.

Instead of blaming yourself, you should be blaming them. You, I, and everyone who has been taken for a ride on the weight-loss merry-go-round were set up to fail. The 5 percent of people who succeed in weight-loss programs are those who would succeed anyway. A friend of mine lost thirty pounds on Weight Watchers and has kept it off. However, she would have done it no matter what program or over-the-counter system she used.

Just like the sweet-talking bastard who has no intention of sticking around after he sticks it to you, the majority of these weight-loss peddlers have no intention of teaching you how to flip off your fat switch. Just like the bad boy who dumped you and then slithers around to make up, they rely on you blaming yourself for failing.

Corporations exist to make money. That's their first priority. They know that by restricting how much you eat, you will lose weight. They know the odds are stacked in their favor that you will recycle through their programs more than once. They make money. You lose money. More important, you might lose your health.

Weight Watchers (*Or whatever name it's going by this year*)

In 1963, Jean Nidetch, the founder of what was to become Weight Watchers, met with friends in her home with the intention of offering support and accountability. That simple formula and small group worked without the corporate greed attached. I don't believe she would think much of the company today.

"Everything is on the menu. 200+ zero Points® foods you never have to portion or track." This come-on hooks us at hello. We can eat pizza and hamburgers, chimichangas, bacon, and chocolate chip pancakes. They advertise that we can *"Eat what you love!"* and still become healthy.[3] Really? The foods we love are the reason we're here in the first place. And they know it. According to the Weight Watchers' business plan, keeping clients coming back, even for decades, *is* good business.[4]

This company changes its programs as often as some people change their underwear. The Freestyle program—its most recent as of this writing—tells you not to worry. Now you can eat two hundred free foods, including eggs, chicken, lentils, beans, fruits, and most vegetables. All you want. Just monitor yourself. That's like telling an alcoholic to have just one shot of whiskey. How convenient. If we fail, which you will and which I did more than once, it's our fault. With one hand, they reel you in with promises, and with the other, they wave away responsibility for the results.

Let's look at fruit as a zero-point food. Have a banana. They're loaded with potassium, fiber, and are fat-free. A medium one contains about 110 calories and thirty carbohydrates. That's a lot of carbs and calories to offer as a free food. If you're concerned with this concept, Weight Watchers has a handy answer. According to its website, "If you're overeating bananas because they're 'free,' you might want to pull back a bit."[5]

How? Overeating the foods Weight Watchers now counts as zero-points guided me into an ass wider than the seat cushion on a chair-and-a-half. Our hunger for food is only a symptom of what we're really hungry for, and until we discover and deal with the causes, we will never be able to "pull back a bit."

Weight Watchers frozen meals and snacks further fuel our cravings. The Smart Ones Chicken Oriental is 71 percent carbs. The Dark Chocolate Nut Breakfast Square is 59 percent fat. This isn't the kind of food that helps curb your appetite for long. They even have thousands of recipes that members can make at home. The catch is that you have to make sure you don't binge on your favorite homemade lasagna or macaroni and cheese or pineapple upside-down cake—a feat that is nearly impossible when you are already out of control.

One constant about Weight Watchers is change. The leaders and receptionists I interviewed during the last year (they were called that until 2018, but today they are called wellness coaches) told me that the company trots out a new program every year. Each fall, employees throughout the country go through the annual training, where they watch a video touting the latest plan and explaining why it's so much better than last year's. Before these and all training sessions, leaders and receptionists are weighed because a high percentage of them are flirting with being over the goal weight they are required to maintain. Guess the program doesn't work any better for the employees than it does for us.

Although Weight Watchers is now attempting to shed its dated moniker by referring to itself as WW, and is calling its centers "studios" and its leaders "wellness coaches," nothing has changed—not the meeting rooms, not the cheerleaders in charge, not the product sales—nothing except for the fact that you don't need this program by any name.

Although Weight Watchers requires its members to weigh in only once a month, most step on the scale every week before the meeting. As I stood in line, the other women and I would exchange stories about our progress while pawing through the snacks and candies on the product shelves. If it was a bad week, I'd hear, "There was a party," or "We went out to dinner, and I couldn't resist," or everyone's excuse when none other is available, "I was bad." This one was always accompanied by a small shrug and foolish grin. Sharing our confessions helped us to feel a little less guilty about what we knew was coming. I used each of those excuses and more. At the bottom of each was the truth. I was obsessed with food. We all were, and this program was helping us stay hooked.

I joined and left Weight Watchers three times, each time thinking I was the failure. The last time I signed up, I recognized many of the same faces I'd seen before. Sitting there like Saturday night sinners testifying at a Sunday-morning revival meeting, they made their confessions.

"I ate a whole bag of Cheetos."

"I had three helpings of enchilada casserole."

Today, some of Weight Watchers' frozen meals claim to be heart-healthy. However, the Smart Ones line is still full of GMO ingredients, and most meals contain preservatives. But any appearance of helping you get healthy is negated by this insane idea of Freestyle eating. If you can eat two hundred free foods, why pay? Instead of plunking down your hard-earned cash for another round of the lose-and-gain game, think about what you like about the program.

Despite the mind-boggling amount of free foods, they still encourage members to track what they eat. I agree. I've always lost more consistently when I take the time to track my food. You don't need Weight Watchers for this. After reviewing fifteen studies relating to dietary self-monitoring either with a paper diary or electronically, the National Institute of Health reported there are, "significant associations between self-monitoring and weight loss."[6] You can find many free apps that track food, exercise, and weight. MyFitnessPal, Lose It!, and SparkPeople are just a small sample of what's available.

Nevertheless, what may work for you is a controversial subject, especially when connected to children. Weight Watchers also offers a tracking app called Kurbo aimed specifically at children between the ages of eight and seventeen. The app's traffic light system divides foods into green/healthy, yellow/eat in moderation, and red/limit the amount eaten. You can also purchase video coaching sessions for sixty-nine dollars per month that are supposed to help your child stay on track. Although Weight Watchers claims this app makes losing weight fun and easy for kids, the National Eating Disorder Association disagrees. Thinking of food as either good or bad can lead to guilt and shame if they eat more bad food than allowed. Because of children's developing bodies, leaving their health and eating habits to a food tracker instead of personal monitoring by a health professional could lead to a lifetime of "weight cycling and poor body image." As overweight adults, we have already cycled through many programs and have a poor body image. Do we want our children to suffer the same way?[7]

If weekly meetings aren't helping, now you can get personal digital coaching for an additional fee. Weight Watchers' certified coaches are usually recruited from the membership (the same way as its meeting leaders) and require no skill other than wanting to work for the company. They are trained in "technical skills," which include selling products as well as cheering on members and offering suggestions to stay on track. If you have someone with whom to share your successes and discuss your setbacks, you will do as well or better than you would with Weight Watchers. If you need more in-depth help, find a certified wellness coach who isn't on the payroll.

Nutrisystem (*Expertise from a vacuum cleaner salesman*)

In 1971, thirty-four-year-old vacuum salesman Harold Katz was looking for another job. He had floated from working in his father's grocery store through a variety of sales jobs. Inspired by his mother's yo-yo dieting, Katz decided to go into the weight-loss business. His first attempt at selling liquid protein served by a staff of doctors and nurses working at storefront "medical" centers resulted in some fatal heart attacks in crash dieters. In 1977, with the help of a microbiologist, he revamped the company, calling it Nutrisystem, and by 1982, it was worth $300 million but in financial trouble. Enter Donald McCulloch, former marketing vice president who had developed the Pan Pizza at Pizza Hut, who turned the company around, kicking Katz out in the process. Under McCulloch's leadership, Nutrisystem promised rapid weight loss. Lose they did, and fast. Too fast.

In the early 1990s, more than seven hundred lawsuits were filed against Nutrisystem as clients across the country began developing gallbladder disease from losing weight too quickly. By 1993, the company was bankrupt again. But that didn't stop the beast from lurching back to life. Like Dr. Frankenstein, the next boss, Michael Heisley, specialized in reviving dead businesses. He kept selling the food at the centers and added Nutrisystem Rx, a pharmacy-like branch that pushed the latest fad, a deadly combo of fenfluramine and phentermine—fen-phen. The drugs helped people lose weight, but also caused blood to leak back into the heart valves because the heart was no longer beating efficiently.[8] That lid blew, and the public found out about the heart valve damage this toxic concoction caused. Hello, lawsuits. Goodbye, weight-loss centers. Did the creature die? Nope. It morphed into an online-only program that still delivers food to your door.[9]

In 2018, the company sold to Tivity Health Systems in Nashville for $1.4 billion. The giant is headed by CEO Dawn Zier, an engineer and marketing whiz who is responsible for the Fast 5, Turbo 10, and Lean 13 campaigns—all wildly successful money-making plans. Nutrisystem is a testament to the endurance of the direct sell and the gullibility of its clients, who shell out thousands of dollars for its food.

Nutrisystem promises "No fads. No gimmicks." No, just chemical shakes and frozen meals and snacks loaded with fat, carbs, and sugar. Better get a second job to pay for this expensive plan. Sure, it's convenient to have meals delivered. However, at $240 to $390 per month for one person minus the cost of fresh fruit, vegetables, and dairy, this program can be a budget-buster.

While these food products are no better than their competition, Nutrisystem is convenient. You choose the shakes, food, snacks, and desserts you want, and they deliver it right to your door. No thinking required.

Yes, most of the frozen meals are fewer than 300 calories, but most of the calories come from carbs and fat. The Meatloaf Sandwich is 55 percent carbs. Although the Artichoke & Spinach-stuffed Chicken Breast is high in protein at 37 percent, it's also 45 percent fat.

The ingredients list for the Turbo Shakes reads like a science experiment. These concoctions contain various chemicals that are supposed to build muscle and encourage weight loss but often give you diarrhea.[10]

You like the convenience of pre-made food; otherwise, you wouldn't have signed up for this home-delivery service. But why not make it yourself? You can prepare a week's worth of lunches ahead of time. Quinoa, lentils, and beans make great salad bases. Try hummus and vegetables or fruits and nuts for snacks. Get the family involved too. Sending your kids to school with a nutritious lunch they helped prepare teaches them healthy habits and gives them better options than the cafeteria or snack bar. Chances are if you're overweight, so is your spouse or partner, and they will benefit as well.

You'll have the advantage of choosing unprocessed, fresh, and healthier ingredients without the chemical additives of Nutrisystem's meals while saving yourself a bundle of money.

Jenny Craig (*If you've got the cash for this, you can afford real food.*)

This multi-million dollar organization began in 1970 when entrepreneur Sid Craig bought a failing chain of fitness clubs in New Orleans and hired then Jenny Bourcq to help run them. By 1979, they were married, and Body Contour was earning $35 million annually. Not bad for a former dental hygienist and a dance instructor who owned five Arthur Murray franchises. A few years later, they sold the fitness clubs to Nutrisystem and headed to Australia, where Jenny Craig, Inc. was born.[11]

After a two-year non-competition clause expired, the Craigs headed back to the United States and soon left Nutrisystem eating their dust. Then the company's progress started to resemble a fire sale. In 2006, they sold Jenny Craig, Inc. to Nestlé for $600 million. In 2013, Nestlé sold it to North Castle Partners, LLC, former owners of Atkins. Getting dizzy from the corporate merry-go-round? You should be. Superficially, they reel us in with promises of let-us-handle-your-life, but their bottom line is all about profits.[12]

Jenny says, "We give you everything you need to succeed. With us you don't have to count, track, or worry about what you eat."

If you don't mind cashing in your retirement and spending between six thousand and eight thousand dollars a year per person, excluding fresh fruits, vegetables, and dairy, in order to eat their version of over-priced, over-processed food, this might be the plan for you.

Although some people may think that a high price equals better results—and this one brags that its members lose three times the weight as those on other plans—its long-term failure rate is identical to Weight Watchers and Nutrisystem, and the food is not nutritionally superior.

In reading the labels of several Jenny Craig meals, I discovered these products to contain additives, artificial flavors, added sugar, and hydrogenated oils (trans fats). Vegetables, when there are any, are near the bottom of the list. Out of twenty-eight dinners, sixteen are pastas with cheese, cream sauces, or both. Like Nutrisystem, all Jenny's entrees have fewer than 300 calories. I also calculated the nutrition value ranges and found them to vary from 17 to 19 percent fat and 38 to 64 percent carbohydrates.

Their latest hype is a DNA test to determine the best plan for their customers. Researchers at the Stanford University School of Medicine disagree. Led by Christopher Gardner, PhD, a recent study focused on whether either insulin or genetics affected weight loss. In February 2018, the Stanford Medicine News Center reported, "Neither option is superior." The study further found that cutting either carbs or fats results in losing weight in about the same proportion, and that neither insulin levels or genotype patterns can predict success on either diet. Save your money on this one.[13]

Like Weight Watchers, Jenny Craig has centers, but the meetings are private and one-on-one with a counselor. Another thing that sets Jenny Craig apart is the way they push their clients. A former counselor I interviewed said, "I felt like a telemarketer." Try to leave the center without buying your next week's food supply because you can't choke down the stuff you already have and you're subjected to the *leftover food dialogue,* which is basically a shaming technique about cheating on your diet. Call to cancel or reschedule an appointment and you'll receive the *reschedule call dialogue,* designed to shame you into showing up no matter what your excuse.

"I had a client who wasn't going to be able to come in for over a week because her mother passed away," the ex-consultant said. "I was told to call her daily."

Another ex-employee I talked with admitted that she would never eat the food herself because it was too "chemically laden." No kidding.

Overweight people pile enough shame on their own heads without having to be subjected to it by the people they hire to help them.

Even most of Jenny's long line of celebrity spokespersons fail, and none more spectacularly than Kirstie Alley. From 2004 through 2007, Alley represented the company and lost seventy-five pounds. As soon as she left, her weight began to creep and then rocket upward until she gained back every ounce.[14] Fast-forward nine years to 2014, and she signed on again, replacing Valerie Bertinelli. The press release stated, "We hope Kirstie's return as our ambassador will provide continued encouragement for our members who...are looking for a program that works." Works? Give me an effing break.

It didn't work for Kirstie—twice. Although she lost fifty pounds this go-around, as soon as she left, she began to yo-yo again.

Nor did it work for Valerie Bertinelli. During the seven years she was Jenny's celebrity shill, Bertinelli lost and kept off forty-five pounds. Less than a year after her ties with Jenny Craig ended, she had regained at least fifteen pounds. Although Bertinelli blamed it on a broken foot and doctor's orders to rest, I wondered why she couldn't have used the healthy-eating habits she must have learned while working for Jenny Craig. Or why she didn't order a supply of food to eat while recuperating. Or why she couldn't call one of those dedicated personal consultants for help. A year later, when I read that Bertinelli had told *Entertainment Tonight* she was through checking her scale, I knew she had fallen off the health wagon.[15]

Today, her *Valerie's Home Cooking* show on the Food Network supposedly puts a new and healthy spin on traditional comfort food. She is also a judge, along with celebrity baker Duff Goldman, on *Kids Baking Championship*, where some of the child contestants are already overweight.

For the money you lay out on this processed food, you could enroll in a home delivery meal service and still have cash left over for a vacation. Services such as Purple Carrot, Hello Fresh, and Blue Apron deliver meal kits in a variety of food plans, including ones that focus on weight loss and are plant-based. Most require less than an hour to prepare, and all contain everything from the main ingredients to the spices. You still don't have to grocery shop or think about what's for dinner. Even better, you don't have to worry about additives, freshness, or whether you need to choose between eating and paying the rent.

In contrast, these big three weight-loss programs have not worked for so many people. They keep you hooked on unhealthy food, while taking your money and your self-respect. Don't fall for their carefully targeted ads. Take charge of your own body, starting now.

CHAPTER 9

THE GREAT AMERICAN MEDICINE SHOW

In the late nineteenth century, the traveling medicine man with his wagonload of patent medicines provided entertainment and a variety of cure-alls to the American public. Newspapers and magazines were crammed with ads for miracle medicines and devices that promised to heal anything that ailed you.

Swallow the Rainbow

By the 1900s, bizarre ways to lose weight were evolving as fast as the junk-food market. As the population grew fatter, the scammers grew richer. The medical profession didn't help. To the contrary, during the 1940s, the American Medical Association approved the sale of amphetamines Benzedrine and Dexedrine for weight loss. By 1949, people were shelling out $7.3 million on these little speed bombs.

Diet doctors and weight-loss clinics were buying direct from diet pill manufacturers and making a killing in profits. The pills were so cheap to manufacture that these doctors could purchase 100,000 amphetamine tablets for seventy-one dollars, and then sell them to patients for as high as $12,000.[1]

Widespread distribution of Benzedrine tablets had started in World War II when the government dispensed them to the military as mood boosters. The uppers kept the troops in combat longer and supposedly helped prevent "combat fatigue," the forties term for PTSD. By the end of the war, when we didn't need to drug the military any longer, Smith, Kline & French, the pharmaceutical company that made Benzedrine, changed its focus to weight loss. Soon, a whole generation of women became hooked on what were then called rainbow diet pills. The colors didn't matter. The combinations were the same: amphetamine and a barbiturate to control the jitters and irritability. These combinations of uppers and downers were marketed directly to thousands of diet-clinic physicians, who prescribed them freely to anyone who wanted to lose weight. Although the Food and Drug Administration and the American Medical Association outwardly disapproved of this drug free-for-all, another twenty years passed before the government finally cracked down. By that time, several young women had died, and 3.2 million Americans were hooked on what was basically prescription speed.[2]

As the population continued to get fatter, and undaunted by the new restrictions against pushing diet pills, the medical profession found new ways to stay in the weight-loss business. In the 1972, Dr. Robert Atkins wrote *Dr. Atkins' Diet Revolution* and started a popular trend of eating a high-fat, low-carb diet. In April 2003, Dr. Atkins died from slipping on an icy sidewalk and hitting his head. However, according to an article in *The New York Times*, he may have been a victim of his own diet. In what the city medical examiner's office called, "a mistake," details of Dr. Atkins' medical report were released. The report concluded that

Dr. Atkins had "a history of heart attack, congestive heart failure, and hypertension."[3]

During the eighteen years I worked in an acute care hospital, I saw doctors who saved patients every day who couldn't save their own lives because they were just as addicted to food and suckered in by the latest fad as I was. Even after the Atkins news, one of the cardiologists on staff at the hospital where I worked insisted the diet wasn't harmful. One day, he walked into the office with a plate full of bacon he'd purchased in the cafeteria. "This is the best diet," he said. "No carbs." No nutrition either—just fat, nitrates, and preservatives.

A doctor friend pushed Medifast at me, even as his belly protruded from his white coat. He also profited from selling the Medifast diet plan and products, which doctors still do today. A website aimed specifically at physicians says, "OPTAVIA offers you an opportunity to transform your practice while creating more autonomy and potential revenue, free from the constraints of managed care."[4] Don't think this is anything special. You don't have to be a physician to sell OPTAVIA, the new name for the direct-marketed subdivision of Medifast. The plan is promoted to anyone who wants to sell its products and earn a commission. This version includes an individual coaching option along with its diet plan, but don't assume that means getting help from an actual health coach or nutritionist. Most coaches are recruited from the customer base, just as Weight Watchers does.

Regular Medifast, which you can buy online, offers two diet plans. Medifast Go! is the original diet of 800 to 1,000 calories a day that puts you in starvation mode for a quicker weight loss. Customers are required to eat five of the Medifast meal replacements daily, as well as one meal of lean meat, fish, or poultry, and vegetables, or "real food" as the website says. Medifast products—shakes, bars, and the usual pasta dishes, including macaroni and cheese—are low in calories but filled with processed ingredients and high in fat and carbs. The vanilla meal replacement shake is 47 percent carbohydrates. You'll lose weight, but the hitch is transitioning back to regular food. This is where most people fail. Once you return to eating real food, the weight piles back on because this diet does nothing to help you overcome your obsession with sugar, fat, and carbs. The less strict version lets customers eat more real food from the start and less of its processed products for a slower loss. Neither plan has long-term success. This stuff didn't work for the doctor who tried to sell the program to me any better than it does for the majority of people who buy it. The last time I saw him, he was fatter than ever. Sound nutrition in the form of a whole food, plant-based diet is too simple a fix for the majority of the medical profession to consider.

Even our hospital's nutritionist was obese. Here was someone who had studied nutrition and still couldn't maintain a healthy weight. The cafeteria food didn't help anyone, including me, who ate there every day. The steam tables held a variety of comfort foods, ranging from mashed potatoes and gravy to meatloaf and enchiladas. You could get pancakes and French toast for breakfast, as well as an assortment of doughnuts and pastries. A separate grill served meat-stuffed sandwiches, burgers, and pizza. If you wanted to eat healthier, your choices were limited to a few pre-made salads and whatever vegetable was offered at the steam table.

React Instead of Prevent

Get sick. Get a pill. Get surgery. Get diagnosed with a life-threatening illness and be subjected to a variety of treatments, all designed to attack the disease. The practices of preventive and integrative medicine are still not included in mainstream medical practices, and insurance companies would rather pay thousands for your hospital stay than a couple of hundred dollars for preventive tests and treatments. If you fell over at work—which one of our physicians did with a heart attack—you could get help fast. Even in a hospital setting, the prevailing attitude was reactive in taking care of diseases after they happened, not proactive in helping people prevent illness.

After you've tried everything and still can't lose, there's always a bariatric surgeon handy who's sharpening a scalpel and waiting to slice-and-dice away that fat. If you think that having your stomach surgically reduced to the size of a thumb is the one true magic cure-all for weight loss, think again. Just as every other weight-loss method, bariatric surgery has a failure rate that should make you think twice before resorting to this solution. According to the Mayo Clinic, only 7 percent of patients have maintained at least a 10 percent weight loss after twelve years.[5]

If you are afraid of having most of your stomach removed, don't worry. You can have your fat sucked out with liposuction, and you don't need a specialist. Your internist, general surgeon, dermatologist, or plastic surgeon can take a course and be approved. If you don't like the idea of having a laser and vacuum tube stuck in your body, you can freeze your fat away with CoolSculpting. Of course, none of these techniques work any better than the others because the bottom line is that you always regain the weight if you don't change your lifestyle.

Doctors are taught how to prescribe blood pressure and cholesterol medications to treat fat-clogged arteries. Coronary artery disease is virtually nonexistent in populations who consume plant-based diets. When patients with heart disease switch to a plant-based diet, more than 80 percent show improvement in lowering cholesterol and cleaning their arteries without further drugs or surgery.[6]

Physicians pump patients full of insulin, and then amputate after diabetes has destroyed the circulation to a toe or leg. With proper nutrition, most patients who lose weight lose their Type 2 diabetes.

According to the Harvard School of Public Health, despite the fact that an estimated 50 to 80 percent of chronic disease is affected by nutrition, only about one-fifth of American medical schools require students to take a nutrition course. Most of those courses require less than twenty-five hours of instruction. Medical students aren't taught preventative medicine. Instead, the focus is on treatment after the disease appears.[7]

When these programs and fixes fail, you go to another doctor. They can't help because they aren't any better at staying healthy than you are. A study by the National Institute of Health revealed that 40 percent of physicians are overweight and 23 percent are obese. In addition to harming their health, obese and overweight doctors were less likely to feel confident in counseling their own overweight patients. This is partly because the doctors worried their patients wouldn't take them seriously. Why should we?[8]

A well-respected, obese oncologist I knew regularly ordered a chili dog with fries from our hospital cafeteria. He spent his retirement years in and out of the hospital with multiple surgeries for stomach cancer. When it comes to long-term health, doctors are as unhealthy and uninformed as most of us. When you rely on people who can't take care of themselves, how do you expect them to help you take care of yourself?

Get Inside Advice

Physicians may be reluctant to talk to patients face-to-face and not know anything about nutrition, but they are happy to churn out diet books by the truckloads. Today, there are more than one thousand diet books on Amazon written by doctors. Each book promises some secret knowledge this or that physician has discovered after years of research.

Dr. Arthur Agatston's popular book, *The South Beach Diet,* rolls out its plan in three phases. Phase 1 cuts out almost all carbohydrates which is supposed to "reboot" your metabolism. This phase drastically cuts calories, so you see your weight begin to drop. In Phase 2, you start adding carbs again, and by Phase 3, you're supposed to have learned how to eat healthy and reached your goal weight. While this plan does emphasize healthy eating, the catch is that there's no proof at all that you will lose weight, and the long-term results are just the same as every other diet. If you don't want to do this on your own, you can always buy one of the available programs for about three hundred dollars a month, not including the cost of fresh vegetables and fruits, and have their diet meals delivered right to your door. South Beach sells shake mixes that "blend up just like your favorite fast food shake" and sound about as nutritious. The first five ingredients in the Chocolate Ice Crush shake mix are sunflower oil, cocoa processed with alkali, maltodextrin, calcium caseinate, natural flavor, and modified tapioca starch.[9] Does this even qualify as food?

There are plenty of physician-authored books on nutrition and healthy eating that promote plant-based diets without trying to sell you more over-processed and expensive diet foods. The catch is, they don't promise you anything but how to eat for optimum health. You have to do the work.

Today's weight-loss schemes are certainly slicker and spew more scientific-sounding drivel, but they are nothing more than this generation's version of the traveling snake oil pitchman who hawked elixirs from the back of a horse-drawn wagon. More than a hundred years later, we're fatter than ever.

Take Responsibility

In 2018, more than $329 billion was spent to treat cardiovascular disease and stroke. According to the Centers for Disease Control, about 80 percent of those cases were caused by poor diet, lack of exercise, alcohol, and obesity. Additionally, the CDC, Surgeon General's office, and other public health officials warn that sitting is becoming as life-threatening as smoking.[10]

Obesity and a sedentary lifestyle don't just increase your risk for heart disease and a variety of other deadly diseases. Your immune system suffers too. As bad as that reality is, worse is the fact that preventable illnesses connected to our lifestyles are on the rise, while life expectancy for the average American has been steadily declining. We are literally killing ourselves with food, and the medical profession doesn't offer much help.

A woman I knew was never overweight despite eating a diet heavy in meat, dairy, and processed food. She felt that because she wasn't overweight, she was healthy. Wrong. One day, while taking her morning bike ride, she fell over with a massive heart attack. Over the course of the next year, she had five stents placed to open her blocked arteries and finally decided she should eat more plants. Today, she's on blood thinners as well as medications to control her high-blood pressure and cholesterol levels. She still eats meat and dairy because her doctor told her it is okay.

Another doctor I knew bragged that his arteries were "as clean as a baby's" even though he was probably one hundred pounds overweight. He kept them clean with megadoses of a mix of drugs he self-prescribed. I don't know what else he may have taken for any other obesity-related issues he may have had, but clean arteries or not, his lifestyle wasn't only threatening to him, it set a dangerous example for his patients.

On the other side of that hazardous health coin is a man who has, against all odds, and most of his many doctors' advice, literally pulled himself from a life of near-total paralysis.

As a former Air Force cargo pilot, J had traveled all over the world. He exercised, was not overweight, and considered his diet healthy because he ate no fast food and didn't drink soda. He had no known health issues until the day he suffered a brain aneurysm and had a stroke while undergoing surgery to repair the dissecting artery. When he woke up, he was paralyzed from the neck down.

Although the doctors assured J he would live, they told him it wasn't possible to know whether he would ever walk again. One week post-op, he was moved into a regular room, and then to a rehabilitation facility. Luckily, as his damaged nervous system began to heal, J was able to move his arms and legs and take a few steps with the aid of a walker. He was also in constant pain.

"My whole body had that pins-and-needles feeling you get when your leg goes to sleep," he said. "The slightest touch made my skin feel like it was being torn off." Because his muscles were rigid from the stroke and the nerve damage, he needed therapeutic massage, so his doctors prescribed pain medications so he could tolerate the sessions.

By the time he was discharged and started to continue his therapy as an outpatient, J was taking sleeping pills, pills for depression, pills to help his nerve damage, and painkillers. When he began to walk better, the doctors advised that he get Botox injections in his hamstrings to help lengthen the muscles and, hopefully, help his gait. They recommended slicing the Achilles tendon in his right leg to give it more flexibility. He refused.

"That was when I knew that if I were to get well, I would have to do it myself," he told me. "All the doctors were doing was pushing more and more medications on me. And none of it was helping."

Because he wasn't exercising any longer, he was gaining weight, which made him feel even worse.

So he started educating himself about food. He talked to nutritionists, yoga teachers, and other holistic practitioners. He questioned his massage therapists to learn as much as he could about how the body recovers from injuries such as his. One thing they all agreed on was that the first thing he could do was to switch to a vegan diet. He did.

"Transitioning to a vegan diet was like my body taking in an incredible breath of fresh air. I was taking the poisons out of my body."

His doctor did not agree with his decision to stop the painkillers, sleep aids, and nerve pills. "He especially didn't like hearing that I was going vegan," he laughed. "He acted alarmed that I wasn't eating meat any longer and asked where I got my protein."

Five months later, he was in Paris, "climbing the steps of the Notre Dame Cathedral."

He went back to work as a ground school/flight simulator instructor. Although he still has difficulty walking and suffers numbness and pain throughout his body, J is convinced that changing his diet was the pivot point of his recovery. He swears that if he had not stopped eating processed foods and animal products, he would not have made the astounding progress he's made.

"I know that if I had continued eating the way I did in the past, I might not be dead by now, but I would be sick, probably diabetic, and certainly not able to walk," he said.

No matter how good your doctor is, no matter how cutting-edge the medications, treatments, and procedures he or she prescribes, the ultimate responsibility for your health is yours.

CHAPTER 10

A LEGACY OF POISON

You buckle up your children in the car. You teach them not to talk to strangers. You try to protect them any way you possibly can—except from the food they eat. Like the neighborhood drug dealer lurking near the schoolyard, the food industry pushes its own variety of addictive junk that can be just as life-threatening as any illegal drug.

Targeting Our Children

For decades, the food companies have hired advertising companies to devise ingenious ways to sell us hundreds of overly processed products with little to no nutrition. This Big Food push to gain market shares and keep their profits rolling in often comes to the detriment of our children's current and future health.

Through toy giveaways, cartoon characters on cereal boxes, and movie tie-ins, commercials are specifically aimed at grabbing the attention of children as young as two years old. The industry has used pop stars such as Mya and Common to hawk Coca-Cola to your teenagers. Beyoncé pushing Pepsi and Justin Timberlake's

McDonald's jingle make it look glamorous to drink and eat these nonfoods. Lil Nas X's Doritos and MC Hammer's Cheetos commercials were hits from Super Bowl LIV's advertisements. Celebrities add credibility and glamour to these products. The catch is that we are sacrificing our children's health right along with ours.

Eighty percent of the food and 71 percent of the beverages hawked by celebrities have little or no nutritive value. Children and teenagers are exposed to more than 25,000 television commercials a year that push unhealthy foods. More than ten thousand of those commercials are specifically aimed at kids between the ages of twelve and seventeen. Food ads on television make up 50 percent of the advertising time on children's shows and are dominated by unhealthy products such as candy, snacks, cereals, and fast foods. *Zero* ad time is dedicated to selling fresh fruits and vegetables.[1]

Cereal and snack food companies and fast-food chains spend billions getting kids hooked on their products, and are succeeding.

Harming Our Children

The Centers for Disease Control statistics show that since the 1970s, childhood obesity rates have tripled. Today, one out of five children and teenagers between the ages of six and nineteen is considered obese. Thirty years ago, Type 2 diabetes was considered an adult-only disease because of its direct link to obesity. Today, it is widespread in young overweight adults. Unless their diets change, one-third of the children born after 2000 will develop Type 2 diabetes in their lifetime. Fatty liver disease, once almost entirely limited to older adults, is now the most common liver condition in obese children. Since the 1980s, the rates have tripled in correlation with the rising number of fat kids. All overweight children have a much greater risk of developing heart disease and a variety of cancers.[2] Sleep apnea and asthma have increased. So

84

have polycystic ovary syndrome and menstrual disorders in teen girls. Obese children often have high blood pressure. Hip and knee pain are common because their growing musculoskeletal system becomes damaged from the excess weight.

The food industry's greed and our ignorance are turning even our toddlers into sugar addicts. Three of the first four ingredients in General Mills's Lucky Charms are some form of sugar (Whole oat flour, marshmallow bits, sugar, and corn syrup). Products such as Fruit Loops and Cocoa Pebbles aren't any better. These are just three of a long list of sugar-filled cereals that you may be feeding your children.[3]

We are angered and appalled by people who threaten children. Yet we never connect that intolerance for others who endanger their lives to the ones who sell them substandard nutrition. Instead, we make hits out of cooking competition shows where many of the kid competitors are overweight. Because our own lifestyles neglect nutrition, we are raising an entire generation of children who are programmed from birth to overeat and who possibly have shortened life spans because of the toxic nonfood we've fed them.

Hooking Our Children

The Centers for Disease Control recommends that children between the ages of two and nineteen consume no more than six teaspoons of sugar daily. Yet, the average American kid eats a staggering thirty-two teaspoons of sugar each day. When you stop to think that one eight-ounce serving of breakfast cereal contains an average of three teaspoons of sugar and a twelve-ounce can of Pepsi contains ten teaspoons, it's easy to see how that happens.

Just as in adults, high sugar consumption causes inflammation in children's bodies and brains. However, the damage is worse because they are still growing, and the effects of sugar are quicker and can cause lasting harm. Children and teens who are overweight suffer higher rates of depression, behavior problems, and anxiety. They score lower on cognitive tests and often have difficulty concentrating in school.[4] And they don't get any better nutrition.

You send the kids to school with money for a cafeteria meal, but that's no guarantee they will get nutritious choices or even eat what's provided. Today, your kids can even choose their favorite fast food from chains such as McDonald's, Domino's Pizza, and Taco Bell. The average cafeteria has vending machines that spew out everything from the usual Ding Dongs and sugar-filled granola bars to a variety of sodas and "fruit" drinks.

Failing Our Children

The food they eat isn't necessarily safe either. Although the United States Department of Agriculture oversees the national school lunch program, the *Public School Review* states, "a significant percentage of the millions of pounds of meat consumed by children in the school cafeteria continually fail to meet quality standards imposed by fast-food outlets." The national Child Nutrition Act was created to ensure that lunchroom meals are prepared under sanitary conditions. However, as many as 30,000 schools annually slip through the cracks of this over-extended inspection process. Despite more than two hundred pieces of legislation regulating food nutrition in our schools, four out of five schools still do not meet the current USDA guidelines for the percentage of fat contained in the average cafeteria lunch.[5] The nutrition-poor meals served in America's school lunchrooms doubly impact children from low-income families, as lunch may be their main meal of the day.

In the seventies, the government reduced subsidies, and schools were mandated to break even. Food programs were cut from general funds in favor of books and classroom materials. That's when cheap foods, such as pizza and pasta, were included in school lunches. Now, school food is a reflection of what we see in our larger society. Kids from all socio-economic levels are suffering malnutrition, which emerges as learning disabilities, behavioral disorders, and other chronic ailments. Add to that the unhealthy nutrition they may get at home and as snacks, and you can see why they suffer.

The junk food, fast food, and processed foods you're getting fatter on are the foods that are ruining your child's health. Maybe you're like one of my clients, who felt too rushed to make breakfast for her children and stopped by McDonald's on the way to school. "I treated them to whatever they wanted at the drive-thru," she said. One child ordered a chocolate milkshake. The other ordered hash browns and ketchup.

You may not head to a nearby fast-food restaurant, but maybe you do have a variety of sugar-loaded cereals in the pantry, and the kids make their own breakfast while you're getting ready for work. Or they choose a toaster pastry and wash it down with more sugar disguised as fruit juice.

Overweight people are often always tired. I could barely get ready for work in the morning, let alone think about preparing a nutritious breakfast or lunch for myself or my family. Evenings are no better. All you want to do is flop on the couch. So you perpetuate the obesity cycle by feeding your children the same garbage you're hooked on. They react the same way you do. They are tired, cranky, and always hungry because they are not getting the nutrients their growing bodies need. I know. I did the same thing.

For years at my house, every Friday night was a standing date with anything from cheeseburgers and French fries to pizza to double-stuffed burritos. I called it grease relief. Giving those zero nutrition meals a glib name gave me permission to binge, and Inner Bitch was right there in my head cheering me on. I told myself that one night a week wasn't bad. Only, some weeks the one night off became two or three. At the time, I was so deep in my food obsession that I could not have told you the number.

My home cooking wasn't any better. I'd make spaghetti or slow-cooker barbecued beef or taco meat. Fresh fruit, vegetables, and salads took last place in my refrigerator. My fat-muddled brain thought that cooking only a couple of times a week should have helped me feel less tired and stressed. My body was too busy fighting off the toxins I poured into it to create the energy I needed.

What I did to myself was appalling, but I am mortified that I fed that potentially lethal diet to my growing daughter. My food addiction was as strong as any alcoholic or drug abuser's addiction, because in order to satisfy my cravings, I endangered my child. What are you doing to yours?

Protecting Our Children

One of the best things you can do for your kids is to set an example by taking care of your own health. When you eat a better diet, you will buy healthier food. That one step will automatically boost your child's nutrition.

You could visit your child's school and see what it serves for lunch. Talk to other parents and teachers. Join a group that advocates for healthy food and safe handling and cooking practices in our schools. Although the government has passed legislation to serve a more nutritious variety of foods, what is actually served is largely left up to each individual school district.

Maybe you could get up a few minutes earlier and prepare your kids and yourself a healthy lunch. Or do it the night before. Let the kids choose what they want from more nutritious options. Fresh fruit cups with berries and slices of apple or banana are easy to make. Instead of traditional peanut butter and jelly, try almond or cashew butter with sugar-free jam on whole-grain bread. Vegetable wraps with hummus, baby carrots, and grapes are quick and nutritious snacks. Prepare several container lunches or salads together once a week. Then all they, and you, have to do is grab one as you leave home in the morning. Look in the recipe section for some easy ideas.

What is hindsight for me can be a way to save your child from the effects of a poor diet.

CHAPTER 11

OBESITY AND
FOOD ADDICTION

Food is a subtle, seductive killer. Overweight people don't get pulled over for steering with their knees while shoving a double cheeseburger in their faces. No one ever called the police because I stuffed myself with three helpings at dinner, and then later fell on the couch in a food-induced stupor. No one ever forced me to check into a fat farm because I ate stale Halloween candy that had been hardening on the floor of my pantry for six months.

Do you hear food calling to you from the pantry or fridge? You know how that last slice of leftover pizza seems to get right inside your head until you can't concentrate on the game show you're watching or the book you're reading or the text you're writing? It would often happen to me. If I imagined the leftover dinner in the refrigerator or the ice cream in the freezer or some other treat in the pantry, that image grew in my head until I saw nothing else and I had to have it.

Food Addicted

At any time, an average 50 percent of the population has some sort of unhealthy relationship with food, and 49 percent of Americans are on a diet. Unfortunately, this latter figure has dropped from 66 percent in 2014. Some of the reasons for this drop in trying to lose weight may include more people who give up because of repeated failures, or physicians and other health care providers who may be reluctant to discuss the subject of weight with patients.[1]

I've felt the embarrassment that others I've talked to feel about not being able to stop eating. One woman said that she just didn't seem to want to lose weight and have better health. She was ashamed of feeling that way about herself but could not get motivated to give up the sweets she loved. I've also felt that way. Maybe you make jokes about your cravings for sweets or fried foods to hide your embarrassment as you keep eating. I've done that too.

Oprah once said that her "drug of choice" was potato chips.[2] I understand what she meant, because I feel the same way about how food has affected my life. But is overeating a true addiction? Probably, at least concerning sugar and heavily processed foods. According to Dr. Nicole Avena, a neuroscientist and expert in the fields of nutrition, diet, and addiction, "When you eat something loaded with sugar, your taste buds, your gut, and your brain take notice. This activation of your reward system is not unlike how bodies process addictive substances such as alcohol or nicotine. An overload of sugar spikes dopamine levels and leaves you craving more."[3]

A study from the University of Michigan reinforced those ideas. Participants in a two-part study worked with the Yale Food Addiction Scale, which is based on standard criteria for substance dependence. That analysis revealed that highly-processed food may trigger addictive responses in the same way as drug abuse.[4] The research team created a list of the twenty most addictive foods. The top five were chocolate, cookies, ice cream, potato chips, and the undisputed, number one champ, pizza. Each food on the list triggered my cravings, and probably trigger yours too.

What's wrong with this picture? The most popular weight-loss programs on the market tell you that you can eat everything on that list and still lose weight. Sure you can, because you're forced to control your portions while on the program. Once you're on your own again, that siren song of cheese-dripping pizza or fudge-swirled ice cream begins to loop through your brain. We can't resist, and the diet industry knows it. Instead of teaching you how to avoid the foods that ruin your health, it makes you dependent on its versions of the same unhealthy food. You're taught that you can't get along without its programs. The truth is that if you get healthy, those programs won't make money.

It seems sugar may also be even more addictive than cocaine. A 2007 study published by the Public Library of Science (PLOS One) and featured in an article from the National Institutes of Health, "the intense sweetness can surpass cocaine reward, even in drug-sensitized and addicted individuals." Sugar hits the same reward centers in the brain that cocaine does, although the downward spiral your body is going through can take years before you see the harm.[5]

My own health had begun to suffer from years of food abuse. My blood pressure was borderline high, my joints ached, and I had trouble climbing one flight of stairs without losing my breath. Reading these studies reinforced what I already knew. If I wanted to lose weight, I had to dump the over-processed, chemical-laden foods. So do you. Dump refined sugars. Dump the pizza. Most important, dump the diet industry because of the ways it contributes to ruining your health.

No Comfort in Comfort Food

Experiments in humans show that for some people the same reward and pleasure centers of the brain that are triggered by addictive drugs like cocaine and heroin are also activated by food, especially those full of sugar, fat, and salt. Like addictive drugs, these foods trigger feel-good brain chemicals such as dopamine. Once people experience pleasure associated with increased dopamine transmission in the brain's reward pathway from eating certain foods, they quickly feel the need to eat again. The reward signals from highly palatable foods may override other signals of fullness and satisfaction. That helps explain why when we say we're chocoholics, we're not far off.[6]

Researchers at Yale University's Rudd Center for Food Policy and Obesity developed a questionnaire that could help identify food addiction in people. The questions addressed behavior patterns and a person's emotional relationship with food. At times, my eating behaviors matched those described by the questionnaire.

- I've eaten much more during the day than I promised myself I would.
- I've eaten to the point of feeling ill, and kept eating when I wasn't hungry.
- I've made a special trip to the store, even late at night, because I wasn't able to wait until the next day for a snack I craved.
- After overeating, I sometimes felt guilty and depressed.

These behaviors show we can lose control over our eating habits and spend almost all of our time thinking about food. Often,

I'd plan my next meal as I was clearing the dishes from the one I'd just eaten. Like people who are addicted to drugs or gambling, people who may be addicted to food have trouble stopping their behavior, no matter how many times they try.[7]

We live in a world of instant gratification, driven by clever marketing aimed at the concept of making our lives easier but solely focused on how much money the food industry can rake in. We're bombarded with food commercials. There's a fast-food restaurant on nearly every corner. Shopping centers and malls are filled with restaurants. You can get anything you want delivered. You can pick up dinner, eat lunch out, and even grab breakfast at the gas station.

Early one morning as I was filling my gas tank at the corner convenience store, I saw a parade of people coming out of the place, each starting their day with some type of nonfood filled with sugar or caffeine or both. I watched as a man and a middle-school-aged boy came out, each carrying a large slushy. Next, a woman wearing what appeared to be health-care worker scrubs walked out the door holding a bag of chips and an energy drink. Two young men dressed in work boots and baseball caps each carried a cup of coffee and a doughnut back to their pickup. The steady stream of people moving in and out of the little store reminded me of a never-ending line of ants that have just found a particularly huge pile of sugar.

We're urged to eat everything we can cram into our mouths. Then, when we're sick or unable to walk across the room without panting, we panic and rush to the doctor or to join the nearest weight-loss program. The doctor treats our symptoms. The weight-loss companies either feed us less of the poison we're hooked on or offer us insanely weird ways to lose. One theory even suggests that if you stick to your diet 80 percent of the time, it's okay to eat whatever you want the other 20 percent. This sounds reasonable. But for me, and maybe you too, eating whatever I wanted 20 percent of the time would soon lead to being right back where I started. Giving up refined sugars and unhealthy processed items does not mean you have to give up enjoying food, including sweets. All you are really giving up are the products that have reduced or eliminated the nutrition by being highly processed. Another diet technique says it's okay to have a free day every week. Stick to your plan for six days and pig out on the seventh. To me, both these scenarios are the same as telling an alcoholic it's okay to get drunk every Saturday night.

Whether overeating is a true addiction, I don't know. I do know that the only way I was able to change the way I ate was by permanently changing the foods I ate. The less processed and fast food I ate, the better I began to feel. The more I focused on plant foods, the less I craved the processed ones. Yes, I had slipups. Yes, I gave up foods I really loved. Cheese was the last to go. Yes, I still have a choice to eat anything I want. But I know what would happen. I would regain probably every pound I've lost, if I didn't drop dead first. I choose to eat a plant-based diet because I know it works.

The only way you can help your body heal is to change your lifestyle, and you are the only person who can make that change. What has happened to you, me, and millions of other people desperate to lose weight is that we have been brainwashed by a hugely competitive industry trying to make as much money as possible. For decades, these companies have told us we can't survive without them, and we've believed them no matter how many times we recycle through their programs.

Think about how many times you've fallen for the marketing hype of a major diet program or tried a new fad because it promised fast and easy results. The fine print always says something like "results not typical" or advises you to eat a low-calorie diet and get more exercise. You don't need to pay for that advice. You already know what it takes.

CHAPTER 12

KNOW WHAT YOU'RE EATING

We love convenience, and the food industry knows how to provide it. We can pick up a pan of frozen lasagna on the way home from work, and then, after kicking off our shoes, pop it in the oven. We can roll through a drive-thru for a sack of tacos, fried chicken, or a double bacon cheeseburger and fries. Thanks to an explosion of food delivery services, we can have anything brought to our door, including the King Kong of fast food, a loaded pizza. This baby has it all: four or five kinds of nitrate-filled meats, a double handful of artery-clogging cheese, and a crust that turns to cardboard after a night in the fridge—if it ever makes it to the fridge. We don't have to think about what we are eating, just what we want and how fast we can get it, except it can often turn into a fatal mistake. These are some obvious health killers, but navigating through the grocery store can be just as hazardous.

You may think that jar of pasta sauce or loaf of whole-wheat bread or any one of a hundred vitamin-enriched, low-fat, zero trans-fat, or sugar-free products is a better choice, but do you know what you're actually eating?

Obesity in America has reached epidemic proportions. According to the CDC, 71 percent of adults and 20 percent of children from age two to nineteen are overweight. Obesity is linked to every disease from arthritis to a variety of cancers.[1]

Want to cut your risk of breast cancer? Lose weight. Fat cells increase estrogen production, and extra estrogen can cause breast cancer tumors to grow. Fat tissue can hide a tumor until it has metastasized throughout your body. Being overweight increases the risk of a reoccurrence.

Competition within the food industry is as fierce as a New York street fight. Food manufacturers spend billions on advertising and marketing to get you to buy their brands. Because they all sell different versions of the same products, getting us to buy what they sell depends on making their boxed stuffing or one-pan dinner mix or chips and snacks appeal to our taste buds. To do this, companies hire a flavorist, sort of like a mad scientist who mixes secret chemical concoctions designed to make us think we're getting authentic food. An article from *The New Yorker* describes these flavorists as, "a kind of secret society. There are fewer than five hundred...in the United States, and they almost never speak about their work outside their laboratories. The consumption of food flavorings may stand as one of the modern era's most profound collective acts of submission to illusion."[2]

Illusion in marketing nonfood to the public isn't limited to flavor. These "natural flavors," along with artificial colors such as FDA-approved Red dye #40, make otherwise colorless and bland fake food tasty and eye-appealing. Red #40 is made from petroleum distillates and has been linked to allergies as well as ADHD in children. This colorful mess contains the toxin p-Cresidine, which the U.S. Department of Health and Human Services says is "reasonably anticipated" to be a human carcinogen.[3] The food coloring has been linked to forty possible side effects. Think about it. Although the FDA has approved Red dye #40, the DHHS warns us that it's probably carcinogenic—two government agencies making contradictory statements about a potentially dangerous artificial ingredient found in everything from cereals to candy to sodas to "strawberry" yogurt that may or may not contain any real fruit. For me, this is all the more reason everyone should stop eating processed food.

Read Every Label

As consumers become more health conscious, the smoke-and-mirror ploys continue with empty promises and dubious health claims that manufacturers slap on their products. Organic, vitamin-enriched, low-fat, sugar-free, and zero trans-fat are a few examples of the labels on everything from breakfast cereal to granola bars to frozen pizza and ice cream. One result of putting these health claims on a package of processed food is that these statements make us think that the calorie content is low.

We see the promise and think we're getting something healthier than the regular version. Wrong. Read the ingredients. The longer the ingredient list grows, the more additives, artificial flavors, and preservatives the food contains. Whatever the product contains the most of is listed first, and the more ingredients it contains, the more highly processed it is.

- Look past the marketing come-on and read what you are really eating.
- Keep the five-ingredient rule in mind. More ingredients equals more additives. If a product has more than five ingredients, you shouldn't buy it.

Another area in which we get conned is the nutrition list. Let's look at your average sixteen-ounce can of Bush's Vegetarian Baked

99

Beans. If you are like I was, all you see is "vegetarian," which equals low calories and healthy. Here is what you get.

The label shows 130 calories, 550 mg of sodium, twenty-nine grams of carbohydrates, and twelve grams of sugar per serving. Sounds reasonable until you realize that one serving is just a half cup. The label lists 3.5 servings in a can. I've never eaten a half cup of beans (or anything else) in my life. That little can has 455 calories, 1925 mg of sodium, 102 carbs, and forty-two grams of sugar. Even if you split it with someone else, you're still getting a high calorie count, and if you eat the whole thing yourself, you'll consume nearly all of the American Heart Association's daily recommended allowance of 2,300 mg (about one teaspoon) of salt and more than the twenty-five grams (six teaspoons for women) or thirty-seven grams (nine teaspoons for men) daily recommended amount of sugar for a very small amount of food. The American Heart Association follows the FDA guidelines for sugar and has set an "ideal" amount of daily salt lower at 1500 mg (a little less than a half teaspoon).[4]

Another clever marketing tactic companies use is to simply label a product "healthy." Conagra Foods' Healthy Choice is a catchy name, but its frozen meals are not necessarily good for you. Take the Sweet & Sour Chicken from the Café Steamers line. At 390 calories, this seems like a good option, until you learn that it's 67 percent carbohydrates, and has 550 mg of sodium. Even its Weight Watchers points equivalent is high at fourteen.

Cut Out Processed Sugar

You might regularly rely on a sweet treat to get you through the afternoon, but I bet the chances are pretty good that you wouldn't snort a couple of lines of cocaine to help you stay awake after lunch. You wouldn't want to end up with rotted teeth or a damaged liver or fried brain or dead. But any of those consequences are exactly what you could suffer if you don't stop eating and drinking sugar.

Over the last one hundred years, our sugar consumption has increased from twelve pounds to more than 120 pounds per year per person.[5]

Until twenty years ago, Type 2 diabetes was considered an adult disease that appeared along with a middle-age weight gain. Today, nearly 45 percent of all cases of diabetes in children and teens are Type 2.[6] Obesity is almost out of control in our children because of their fat-filled diets and sedentary lifestyle. The scariest fact is that the fastest growing group of obese kids is between the ages of eight and ten. If you don't care about what you're shoving down your throat, think about what you are doing to them and their future.

Once you start looking at the labels, you will discover that some kind of sugar is added to almost every processed food, from bread to pasta sauce to even those canned vegetarian baked beans you just read about. The first four ingredients are white beans, water, brown sugar, and sugar.[7] Keep in mind that ingredients are listed in descending order of the amount present according to weight. Basically, this vegetarian chili consists of beans, water, and two forms of processed sugar.

How about your favorite Starbucks beverage? Here's a sample: Venti white chocolate mocha with whipped cream—about eighteen teaspoons, Venti chai tea latte—about thirteen teaspoons, and Venti caramel macchiato—about eleven teaspoons.[8] No wonder we're wired by the time we get to work and want to take a nap before going to lunch.

When you cut yourself or are bitten by an insect, your immune system kicks in and your skin becomes inflamed and tender. When you eat processed foods full of refined sugar, the cells in your body become inflamed, only the inflammation inside you can take decades to cause damage. Your immune system recognizes these refined sugars for the poisons they are and goes into defense mode trying to prevent damage to your body. The deadly catch is that you fuel the damage with every bite of sugar-filled food you eat. So your immune system is cranked on high twenty-four seven, which causes constant inflammation throughout your body. You can stop wondering where your aching joints, bloating, and gas come from. The sugar you're shoving down your throat from obvious sources, combined with the hidden sugars in other foods you eat, is feeding on your body and destroying it cell by cell. The war your immune system is waging with sugar leaves it weakened to fight any outside infection or disease that comes along.

As I discussed earlier, the evidence for treating sugar as an addictive substance is growing. I know that I could never eat just one cookie or one scoop of ice cream or one slice of cake. When I did go on a sugar binge, I walked through the day in a fuzzy-headed haze. I reread notes I'd taken or my to-do list over and over because the moment my eyes left the page, I'd forget what I'd just read. When on deadline, I'd get so anxious that I would write a paragraph, and then jump up to get another handful of cookies or candy from the pantry.

Once I conquered my obsession with sugar, those symptoms went away. Most likely, yours will too. Only don't think that you have to be 122 pounds overweight, as I was, to suffer the consequences of eating sugar-filled foods.

Save Your Brain

The brain needs insulin to thrive, but flood it with refined sugar, and you're flirting with a one-way ticket to the dementia wing of a senior living complex. Recent research shows that Alzheimer's may be another form of diet-induced diabetes. Just as your body becomes insulin resistant when you're overweight, which often leads to Type 2 diabetes, your brain can become insulin resistant from eating too much sugar for too long. People with Type 2 diabetes are already 40 percent more likely to develop Alzheimer's.[9]

A study published in the New England Journal of Medicine shows that even in people without diabetes, above-normal blood sugar is associated with an increased risk of developing dementia. The study concluded that there is a link between dementia and elevated blood sugars in non-diabetic people. The majority of the study participants did not have diabetes. What the researchers found is that *any* incremental increase in blood sugar was associated with an increased risk of dementia—the higher the blood sugar, the higher the risk.[10]

When I was fat, I had an endless supply of sugary treats in my house, my car, and under my desk in my home office so I didn't have to walk to the kitchen for a fix. I had no idea, and didn't care, how much I ate or what I was doing to my body and my brain. All I wanted was the temporary feel-good fix. At my worst, I didn't even taste the stuff. I just shoved it down my throat without thought until I reached the end of the sleeve of cookies or the sack of chocolate and wondered where it had gone.

Our brains have certain automatic appetite-controlling mechanisms that let us know when we've had enough to eat and tell us to stop. Sugar works on these systems differently, keeping us wanting more and more even when we've consumed lots of calories. Sugar triggers the areas of the brain responsible for sensory perceptions that make sweet flavors taste so good and keep us reaching for one more brownie or another bottle of flavored water. My compulsion was obvious, but the hidden sugar in your everyday diet is just as dangerous.

How much sugar do you think you eat? The American Heart Association recommends no more than six-to-nine teaspoons a day. The average person eats twenty-two teaspoons a day.[11] You might not be cramming doughnuts and cupcakes in your mouth, but if you drink vitamin water or eat jarred pasta sauce, you are getting more sugar in your system than you realize. Bread, crackers, barbecue sauce, and instant oatmeal contain added sugars. Even healthy alternatives like nut milks have sweetened varieties.

Even if you think you are watching your sugar intake, you probably do not have any idea of the amount you are really eating. Looking for the obvious sugar, honey, and high-fructose corn syrup is easy. What is harder is learning how the food industry sneaks sugar into processed foods so that even people who are trying to eat healthier are fooled. Additives such as dextrose, maltose, lactose, and dextrin are just fancy names for forms of sugar.

The list of hidden sugars is long. Here are some of the less obvious ones to look for when checking the ingredients list:

- Barley Malt
- Cane juice
- Ethyl maltol
- Fructose (or any ingredient that ends in "ose")
- Fruit juice concentrate
- Maltodextrin
- Mannitol
- Molasses
- Panocha
- Refiner's syrup
- Rice syrup
- Treacle (the British version of molasses)

Eliminating processed foods is the best way to remove the excess sugar from your life. Reading labels is the way to start.

Forget the Soda

One of the worst nonfood scams ever invented is soda in any form. Regular, diet, clear, or colored, these chemical mixes damage your body in every way, from rotting your teeth to increasing your risk of disease. A University of California San Francisco study indicates that drinking a daily twenty-ounce soda ages the skin in the exact same way smoking does.[12]

Soda contains nothing but artificially-flavored water, sugar, and sodium. One can of Coke contains about ten teaspoons of sugar. The added sodium is the reason you're often thirsty for more after the first can or glass. Drinking just two cans of this toxic combo a day can add twenty-six pounds a year to your body. Not only will you have that extra weight to suffer, but soda is linked to heart disease, fatty liver disease, stroke, diabetes, kidney stones, osteoporosis, and pancreatic cancer. Think you're safe with diet soda? The artificial sweeteners in all diet drinks are linked to heart disease and diabetes and can increase the risk of being diagnosed with depression by 31 percent. Oh, and you'll still gain weight.[13]

Along with my miserable eating habits, I literally poured gallons of soda down my throat for years. I even added them to the various diet shakes on the market, including Weight Watchers' mixes on the recommendation of other members and even some group leaders at meetings I attended when a member.

If you did *nothing* but stop drinking soda in all its forms right now, you would sleep better, sharpen your memory, and lose weight as well as cut your risk of becoming ill.

CHAPTER 13

MAKE THE CHANGE

The only hard thing about making a change is making up your mind to start. Think about the last time you really wanted something. Did you save money for a new pair of shoes? Choose to search for a better job? Save for the down payment on a car or special vacation? I bet when you decided what you wanted, you had zero trouble going after your goal. You knew what it took, and you did it. If shoes or a job or a vacation is important enough to make changes for, isn't your life?

Move Your Butt

When I started to exercise, the only thing I could do was walk—make that shuffle. The farthest I could manage was about a half-block from my home. My neighbor, who walked every morning and was far ahead of me on the fitness scale, invited me to join her. I told her that I had "weak ankles" and "bad knees" and probably couldn't go too far, thus giving myself an excuse and easy out. The real reason? I had done little but sit on my rear end for years.

At first, I could make only that half-block before turning around and limping back home. Gradually, that distance stretched to *around* the block, and then to three or four miles a day. From that day until this one, I have kept moving. You can do the same. You don't have to even believe you can succeed. You just have to keep putting one foot in front of the other.

The human body was made to move, not sit and waste away. Exercise doesn't just make you feel better. Moving helps your body clean out toxins and heal quicker. Your body, your mind, and your spirit all will benefit.

Set Sustainable Goals

We are bombarded every day to set goals. Work goals. Relationship goals. Life goals. Retirement goals. Goals are good, but when you concentrate only on the outcome, you can be overwhelmed. Often, when you are obese, your only ambition is to make it to your job or to school or to be able to take care of your family. When you join a weight-loss program or decide to try to lose on your own, that target can be daunting, especially when you are just beginning.

For more times than I can count, every time I set a goal to lose, I always focused on the end goal—those one hundred nasty pounds— which seemed so far away and impossible that I gave up before I started. Setting unrealistic goals is another form of self-sabotage. However, setting the right goals will help you succeed.

- **Choose a measurable goal and be specific.** Instead of saying you'll ride your bike, set a goal of distance or time and how many times a week you will ride. For example: I will take a thirty-minute ride three times a week.
- **Set goals that are attainable.** Make sure your goals fit into your lifestyle. If you can only walk, as I did, when starting

to exercise, then don't buy a pair of running shoes and expect to jog around the block. If you can't get to the gym every day, don't put more stress on yourself by making that a goal. When can you go? What time? How many times per week? Would an online exercise class work for you?

- **Set relevant goals.** Make your goals appropriate to where you are starting from and what's going on in your life right now. As discussed earlier, don't lose for the wrong reasons. You want permanent change, not another setup for failure.
- **Set a time limit.** Deadlines can help you stay on track and motivate you to get started. Be realistic.

Think about the ways you can succeed. When eating in a restaurant, you can substitute steamed vegetables for a loaded baked potato. When buying groceries, you can walk past the chips, sodas, and candy aisles.

Make a grocery list and stick to it. Those end caps and displays at the checkout counter are there to tempt you into impulsively buying something you don't need.

Monitor Your Progress and Reward Yourself

Whether you're keeping a food journal or using a fitness app, monitoring your progress helps keep you accountable. You are the only person who is responsible for either your success or failure. Weighing yourself is part of the process. In the past, anytime I was trying to lose weight, I became obsessed with checking my weight. If I went up a few ounces, I berated myself. If the scale dropped a few ounces, I would be so happy that often I would eat in celebration. Irrational, I know, but that's what happened. The majority of programs suggest weighing only once a week, at the same time each day.

Definitely reward your progress, only not with food. The mental boost will help you remember how good you feel every time you see a lower number appear in the window of the bathroom scale. You will also retrain your brain to disconnect from thinking the only way to celebrate is to eat.

Keep Your Mind and Body Connected

Remember, being mindful is nothing more than the habit of thinking about what you are doing. Practice pausing for a few seconds (about the time it takes to inhale and exhale a deep breath) to think before you blindly reach for a snack or a second or third helping of dinner. Learn to listen to your body. It's smarter than you. Your body knows when it's hungry, and right now, that's about 95 percent less often than you eat. If you pay attention, it will tell you when to feed it and when to keep your mouth shut.

Rely on your spiritual self to help you stick to your goal of getting healthy. Meditation, prayer, and silence all help us to slow down and think about what we do and why. Forgive yourself for the times you had to begin again. You're no longer that person. Learning to connect your mind and body will help you to turn off your automatic response to reach for food as a substitute for expressing your emotions.

Find Support

Having a buddy who will support your battle against food addiction is crucial. Many times, that person is a friend or family or a colleague at work. Sometimes, it's a professional.

My primary buddy is the friend with whom I started walking. She is always supportive and never pressed me to do more or became impatient with my pace while I was losing.

Every overweight person either has an emotional empty place she is trying to fill, or a boxcar of anger she is trying to stuff down with food. Stress, fear, anger, frustration, childhood traumas—all are reasons for over-eating. That old excuse, "I love food," is just an excuse, one I've used many times. I can tell you how I lost the weight, but I can't fix the hole in your life that makes you overeat. You have to do the work on that issue.

What I can do is remind you that you deserve to be healthy. You deserve to be happy. You are as good as anyone else on this planet, and no one has the right to make you feel badly about yourself. Not even you.

Use the Power You Have

Overweight people often feel so powerless that they are almost catatonic. You might think that you can never shed those pounds no matter what you try. You may feel like a failure because you've started and stopped more diets than you can remember. I understand. I've felt the same way, but it's only another lie.

Remember, you have the power to say no to the people who try to push food at you. You have the power to shut up Inner Bitch and take control of your health. You have the power to train yourself to think before automatically reaching for something to eat.

You are not a failure. You are not a slob, pig, or lazy loser. You have been caught in a system that is designed to keep you addicted to food no matter how hard you try or how much money you spend to lose weight. As long as I ate the foods that fed my obsession and bought them from a growing circle of pushers disguised as the weight-loss industry, I had little chance of healing my body. Neither do you.

In addition to dumping the food that's killing you, dump your rabbit food ideas about eating a clean and healthy plant-based diet. No desserts? How about chocolate lava cake, only without eggs, sugar, and flour? Snacks? Try your favorite nuts roasted with maple syrup and cinnamon or cayenne. Main dishes? Everything you eat with meat can be re-created using plants. The internet is crammed with healthy plant-based recipes. Find ones you like, and then tweak them with a variety of ingredients. Experiment with spices and flavors.

In the back of this book are some recipes to get you started. Use them as the beginning of your own investigation into plant-based living. You can check these out and go online and search for recipes for the standards you cook at home. I promise you will be surprised at the variety you find. Besides, it's a much better way to spend your time than posting photos on Facebook of the latest artery-clogging meal you're eating. I ended every food issue I had by moving to a plant-based diet. So can you.

Stock a Plant-Based Pantry

Although putting together a plant-based pantry might seem challenging, you probably already have some basic items. The list below is for your inspiration and to help you to look at plant foods as more than side dishes at dinner. I hope it makes you curious to discover even more plants to try and new dishes to make. I know the steps you're taking now will help your body become as strong and healthy as it can be. Have fun experimenting!

Beans and Legumes

Who doesn't love chili beans or a pot of bean soup on a winter day? Beans and legumes are versatile and cost just pennies a serving. You can eat them cold or hot in soups, salads, as a main or side dish, and so many other ways. If you're like I was, you probably have one or two favorites you keep on hand. Try some you've never eaten, or switch up your standby recipes with a different variety. I stock both dried and canned beans now.

Beans are full of protein and fiber and can help lower blood sugar and cholesterol.

- Black beans
- Kidney beans
- Pinto beans
- Lentils: Lentils are rich in fiber, folic acid, and potassium—all nutrients that aid heart health. With four main categories, red/yellow, brown, green, and specialty (usually black), and several varieties within each category, the flavors, textures, and ways to use them are almost endless.
- Navy beans
- Lima beans
- Cannellini beans
- Great Northern beans
- Chickpeas (Garbanzo beans): Great for hummus, faux tuna salad, and roasting for a crunchy snack.
- Peanuts: Surprised? So was I when I learned there's nothing nutty about these little legumes. Peanuts are a good source of B vitamins, protein, and a variety of minerals.
- Black-eyed peas
- Mung beans: Usually associated with China, mung beans are actually native to India. These nutrition powerhouses are loaded with protein, essential amino acids, antioxidants, and iron.

Grains

Whole grains are high in vitamins, minerals, antioxidants, fiber, and other plant compounds that nourish our bodies and help to prevent disease. Refining grains removes almost all of these nutri-ents by eliminating the bran and germ layers of the grain seed. Milled grains have a finer texture because nothing's left but the starchy endosperm. Products such as white rice, white bread, and white flour have been reduced to simple carbohydrates that act in the same way as sugar. Sure, you get a temporary energy boost, but you get a higher risk for heart disease, diabetes, cancer, high blood pressure, and obesity too. Ditch those gluey grains for hearty ones.

- Quinoa
- Oats
- Brown rice
- Wild rice
- Farro
- Couscous
- Spelt
- Bulgur

Flour

Try baking with flours other than all-purpose white. Here are some of my favorites:

- Quinoa
- Chickpea (Garbanzo bean)
- Almond meal
- Oat
- Whole wheat
- Cornmeal

Nuts

Nuts are one of my favorite foods. Raw are best and most versatile. Full of protein, fiber, vitamins, and minerals, nuts are a powerful

CONFESSIONS OF A FAT COSMO GIRL

source of healthy energy. Most of the fat content in nuts is the healthy monounsaturated and polyunsaturated omega kind. You can eat them raw, make nut milks and other substitutes for anything from sour cream to alfredo sauce, add them to all kinds of baked goods, salads, vegetable and main dishes, or simply roast them for a sweet or spicy snack.

- Almonds
- Cashews
- Filberts
- Peanuts (Technically a legume, peanuts are traditionally included in the nut category, and are inexpensive and nutritious.)
- Pecans
- Walnuts
- Pistachios
- Pine nuts

Seeds and Dried Fruits

Seeds and dried fruits aren't just great for snacks and baking. They can add delicious flavor to whole-grain and vegetable dishes.

- Chia seeds
- Sunflower seeds
- Pumpkin seeds
- Raisins
- Cranberries
- Apricots
- Flaxseed meal: Flaxseed meal is full of omega-3 fatty acids. Combined with a little water, ground flaxseed acts as a binder in baked goods, replacing eggs.

Spices and Herbs

One thing I've had fun with is building a spice collection. My knowledge and experience with spices was pitiful. I barely had the basics. You know, garlic powder, black pepper, table salt, poultry seasoning, cinnamon, and a few other baking spices. Some of those little cans and jars sat in my cabinet for years. Who knew they expired? Not me. When I moved to a plant-based diet and started trying vegan recipes, I discovered a whole new world of flavors.

The herbs I've listed here are the dried versions. Try the fresh ones too. These, and others such as cilantro, mint, and parsley, add a burst of flavor to hot and cold dishes. If you're hesitant to buy a fresh bunch because they don't last very long, you can freeze what you don't use. They will last about a year in the freezer.

You can puree the herbs with a tiny bit of water and pour into an ice cube tray. After the cubes are frozen, empty them into a freezer bag. Or you can remove the stems, and then wash, pat dry, and freeze the leaves. Arrange the leaves in a single layer on a cookie sheet lined with parchment paper until frozen, and then transfer the frozen leaves to a freezer bag. That way, they don't clump together. Label and date the bags.

- Allspice
- Basil
- Bay leaves
- Braggs Organic sprinkle
- Celery seed
- Chili powder
- Chinese five spice
- Cinnamon
- Cumin
- Curry powder

- Dill weed
- Fennel seed
- Garam masala
- Garlic powder
- Ground ginger
- Ground and whole cloves
- Ground nutmeg
- Italian blend (oregano, marjoram, thyme, rosemary, sage)
- Old Bay seasoning
- Oregano
- Poultry seasoning
- Pumpkin pie seasoning
- Ras el hanout
- Rosemary
- Sage leaves
- Salt (pink, sea, kosher, coarse, and fine). Flavored salts are fun to try too.
- Sweet paprika
- Smoked paprika
- Tarragon
- Thyme leaves
- Turmeric
- Whole black pepper

Sweeteners

Pure maple syrup and coconut sugar are the only sweeteners I use.

Oils

A little oil goes a long way. I use very little oil because of having heart disease. Coconut oil has the highest saturated fat content. Canola and other vegetable oils are highly processed and have very little flavor or nutritional value. Sunflower oil is high in omega-6 fatty acids, which can lead to inflammation. The only oils I keep on hand are a good extra virgin olive oil and avocado oil. I use the spray versions and sparingly. Most dishes are perfectly fine with little or no added oil. The less you use, the less you will find you need.

You can substitute applesauce, bananas, pumpkin, or other fruit purees—and even pureed vegetables such as zucchini or carrots—for the oil in many baked items.

Other Suggestions

- **Nutritional yeast:** Full of B vitamins, minerals, protein, and antioxidants, nutritional yeast adds a cheese-like flavor to any food. You can sprinkle it on everything from soup to pasta to salad.
- **Vegetable broth:** Use low- or sodium-free vegetable broth instead of water to add flavor. Tip: Save the trimmings from fresh vegetables in a gallon freezer bag. When it's full, make your own broth.
- **Nut butters:** In addition to our standby peanut butter, a wide assortment of other nut butters lines the grocery shelves. Almond, cashew, pecan, walnut, macadamia nut, and more can be used for anything from salad dressing to vegan cheeses. Nut butters are fun and versatile, but be careful. All are high in calories and fat.
- **Bread:** Ditch the white bread for the whole-grain sprouted kind.
- **Butter and mayonnaise substitutes:** Try mashed avocado or hummus on sandwiches and toast. There are plenty of vegan butter and mayo options. I prefer the soy-free ones. Caution: These are still full of fat.

- **Plant milk:** Trade cow's milk for a plant-based milk. Use only unsweetened, unflavored varieties.
- **Fresh and frozen organic vegetables:** Load up on organic veggies. Try ones you've never eaten. Take advantage of your local farmers' market and its seasonal produce. Buy extra and freeze your favorites.

Appliances, Gadgets, and Other Helpful Tools

- **Instant Pot:** If you don't already have one, this is such a versatile little cooker. You can make anything from soup to stew to desserts to beans. It's a slow cooker and pressure cooker all in one handy machine. Comes in a variety of sizes that will fit any size family and budget.
- **Juicer:** This is one appliance I never thought I would use, but I love having the ability to make my own fresh juice. Tip: Keep the pulp for smoothies and baking. Store in an air-tight container in the refrigerator for a couple of days or freeze for up to two months. You can freeze in ice cube trays, and then pop one or two into a smoothie.
- **Food processor:** Make a chopped salad. Shred potatoes. Make hummus.
- **Spiralizer:** If you prefer spiralized vegetables to ones shredded or julienned in the food processor, then you'll enjoy having this handy gadget.
- **Immersion blender:** I love the convenience of using an immersion blender rather than having to drag out my regular blender to puree soups and vegetables. It is easier to clean and much less work because I don't have to stop to scrape down the sides of the big blender.
- **Nut milk bags:** I use these instead of cheesecloth because unless you're making gallons of nut milk or a huge batch of

vegan cheese, you don't need yards of cheesecloth stuck in a kitchen drawer. Organic unbleached cotton is the best. Make sure the bag is sewn with cotton thread, as nylon threads often break with use and get into whatever you're making. Tip: Keep the pulp for use in baking. Stored in an air-tight container, the pulp will keep in the refrigerator for four or five days. Or you can freeze it for up to a month.

CHAPTER 14

THE TWENTY-ONE-DAY CHALLENGE

During the decades I spent bingeing my way through commercial weight-loss programs, the concept of plant-based eating never entered my mind. Not when food took over my life. Not when I spent the next twenty years cycling through a series of diet failures. After years of refusing to accept that my body was slowly breaking down, I was forced to face my deteriorating health. A series of problems, all within six months, shook me awake to the fact that I was not invincible. All were red flags that my body was flooded with inflammation and my immune system was beginning to crash. Still, I refused to admit it to myself until the day I learned I'd developed coronary heart disease. Only fear could motivate me. There's nothing like thinking you might die to get you off your ass.

That was the day I committed to a plant-based diet. My diet was one vital issue I didn't have to worry about when the pandemic struck. I knew that my immune system was as strong as I could make it because my body was not fighting the effects of unhealthy foods. You can make the same commitment to your own health. I created the Twenty-One-Day Challenge so that you can experience how easy it can be to move to a plant-based diet.

The next twenty-one days are going to come and go whether or not you start taking care of yourself. But instead of finding a new fad to follow and fail at, or gaining another five or ten pounds, why not give yourself and your body a real chance to change?

Keep an Open Mind

Despite my years of excess, moving to a plant-based diet was easier than I had imagined. Anything you cook with meat, eggs, and dairy you can prepare without those ingredients. Once your body is cleansed of the toxins you've poured into it, your palate will change. Remember the first time you tried fat-free milk and cringed at the watery taste? If you stuck with it for a couple of weeks, the flavor of the fat-free version became normal. Then, if you tried whole milk again, it felt thick as cream on your tongue. The same thing will happen when you start eliminating animal and processed products. Artificial flavors will taste artificial. Over-processed items will taste like sugar or salt and little like the food they are supposed to contain.

Moving to a plant-based diet saved my life. I am healthier, have more energy, and feel better than I ever did, even before I was obese. I wish I had made the move sooner. You can start today.

Track What You Eat

Tracking what you eat is crucial. Even the most health-conscious person cannot accurately remember what she's eaten during the day. If you're still mindlessly reaching for food all day, you can't possibly know what or how much you've eaten. Today's apps are sophisticated enough to break down the nutritional values of what you eat so you know how many fat, carb, and protein grams you are consuming.

Every time I tracked my food, I always lost more weight and ate a more well-balanced diet. Today, there are many apps that are compatible across devices and are easy to use, even for non-techie people. All have basic free plans that include a meal planner, tell you the nutrition and calorie count of foods, and provide an exercise tracker. Most allow you to scan a barcode to see the nutrition content on that pound of beans or pasta. You can personalize your daily calorie intake based on how much you'd like to lose and your age, height, weight, and gender. If you choose to upgrade to a paid plan, you can find them priced between thirty and fifty dollars a year.

Cut Out Meat and Dairy

When you stop relying on packaged food, meat, eggs, and dairy, you will be able to make every bite count. You will feel the difference in both your body and your emotions. In addition to the artery-clogging and weight-gain warnings we've all heard about eating meat and dairy products, the animal industry also exposes its customers to other dangers. These industries can expose people to a variety of health-damaging food preservatives, animal hormones, antibiotics, mercury, and other heavy metals, which are toxic to our bodies.[1]

The evidence linking animal products and heart disease is indisputable. Removing animal products from your diet can greatly reduce your chances of developing heart disease—especially if that disease runs in your family as it does in mine.

I grew up on a farm. Although we had plenty of fresh vegetables and fruits all through the year, we ate animal and dairy products, including dessert, every day.

That's not the best diet for someone whose DNA is imprinted with heart disease on both sides of the family. My mother's relatives had no symptoms until they dropped dead, most before age fifty. She died at fifty-five from a heart attack. Although my dad lived to be seventy-nine, he suffered five heart attacks before he reached his seventieth birthday.

Because of my family history, you would think that I would have paid more attention to my own health, especially as I got older. Instead, I avoided the truth on every level. Because I had no visible problems, I told myself I was lucky like my relatives who lived well into their nineties. I simply ignored the facts.

The quote, "Genetics loads the gun, but lifestyle pulls the trigger," has been attributed to several different sources, including Dr. Oz. But no matter who said it first, it's a truth we all should pay attention to. My family health gun was fully loaded with a genetic disposition to coronary artery disease. My lifestyle was spinning the cylinder. At the same time, that lifestyle was causing damage elsewhere in my body, which I also ignored until a series of warnings, all within six months, forced me to think about my health. That's when I decided to see a cardiologist to get a baseline on my heart health. Lucky for me that I made that decision because the test he ordered revealed two partially-blocked arteries. Just as my maternal side of the family, I had no symptoms.

That news finally scared me straight into total plant-based eating. Although I had been slowly eating less meat and dairy, once I realized that my life could literally be in danger, I had no problem dropping the last of those products. There's nothing like thinking you might die to get you off your ass.

How much of your obesity do you blame on your family genes? Maybe you think you've inherited the family fat gene and use that as an excuse. Perhaps you feel destined to get Type II diabetes or develop heart disease or any other disease because it runs in your family. That's not true.

You can't change your genes, but your lifestyle can mean the difference between becoming a victim of your family DNA and living a healthier, longer life.

Cook to Thrive

During the weeks I stayed home during the pandemic, I thought about the stories of family members who had faced the Great Depression and contended with rationing in World War II. I realized their admonishments about cleaning my plate came from their own scarcity of food during those times. I remembered what a doctor had told me years ago about nutrition. "Make every bite count," he'd said. Our bodies need very little of the right kinds of food to thrive. We're conditioned to overeat by clever marketing, advertising, and the fact that there's a restaurant or fast-food place on almost every corner.

In addition to your emotional cravings for food, another reason you overeat is because your body is fighting off the effects of the wrong foods while still craving the nutrients it needs to survive. Say you eat a calorie bomb snack for quick energy, and then an hour later you crash because the sugar high is gone. You're feeling the effects of the sugar addictive reaction, but your body also didn't get the fuel it needed to maintain its energy. Instead of buying more sugar-filled snacks and fast food, think about what you're doing to your body. Even if you do cook most of your meals, are they healthy? Mine weren't. If you're overweight, yours aren't either.

For the next twenty-one days, experiment with new flavors and spices. Try grains and vegetables you've never eaten. I had never tried to cook with lentils and never eaten quinoa. I thought

I hated Brussels sprouts until I had them roasted. I'd never used any flours except all-purpose white flour, or tried substituting maple syrup or coconut sugar for refined brown or white sugar. You can easily learn how to cook plant-based versions of your favorite dishes. I've included some of my favorites in the recipe section to get you started.

What about protein? That's the question everyone asks, and it's the biggest misconception about plant-based eating. Grains, legumes, beans, and plants contain plenty of protein for daily nutrition. Nuts and seeds do too. As with all foods, be aware of the fat and carb contents, but don't worry about getting enough protein from plants. After all, where do you think cows get their protein? From grasses and grains.

What about vitamin B_{12}? Fortified nut and soy milks, soy products, and nutritional yeast are good sources of vitamin B_{12}. Because your body stores this essential vitamin, you can take a supplement once a week if needed.

During those weeks locked inside, I was as frustrated and anxious as anyone I know. I couldn't jump in the car and head to the store for a forgotten item on my grocery list. I couldn't pick up my favorite sandwich or eat out with my loved ones. But I was grateful for the assortment of staples in my vegan pantry. Even with the variety, I was forced to come up with new ways to cook my favorite dishes. I took it as a challenge to experiment with leftovers and different combinations of spices.

You can do that too with most of the items you already have on hand. As you add more plant-based foods to your supply, you'll be eliminating those from animals, and you'll get a bonus. In addition to boosting your health—and depending on how much meat, eggs, dairy, frozen or packaged dinners, fast-food, junk food, pizza delivery, and restaurant meals you buy—you could save a bundle.

Choose Organic

How your food is grown has a huge impact on your health. You might think you're allergic to a certain food, but you may actually be allergic to the fungicides, herbicides, and insecticides sprayed on the crop. Many people find that when they switch to organic foods, their symptoms lessen or, in some cases, disappear. Even if you aren't allergic, the combinations of pesticides used on today's conventional crops have damaging effects on both our physical and emotional health. Don't think washing the produce will solve the problem. The chemicals have been taken up into the root systems through irrigation.

Organic crops in the United States must be grown without synthetic pesticides, GMOs, petroleum-based fertilizers, and sewage sludge fertilizers. Organic farming is safer for the farmers who grow the food and the people who work in the fields. Farming without chemical fertilizers and pesticides is better for nearby birds and animals. Many organic farms are small, local businesses, and the money they earn stays in the community. The food is picked when it's ripe and at the peak of its nutrient value.

Ever wonder why those tomatoes that look so good in the store often are almost tasteless? Commercially grown produce is usually picked green and transported an average 1,500 miles from farm to consumer. Then the fruit and vegetables are often sprayed with ethylene gas to speed ripening before landing in the market.

Glyphosate is the main ingredient in Roundup, the world's most popular weed killer.[2] What you might not know is that commercial farming operations use glyphosate on our food crops, not just to kill weeds, but to desiccate the crop just before harvest. This makes the grain dry faster and more evenly. Glyphosate is regularly used on foods such as oats, wheat, lentils, corn, peas, flax, rye, buckwheat, canola, potatoes, and others. Traces of this poison are found in the processed foods you and your family eat. For example, glyphosate has been found in almost two dozen of General Mills' breakfast cereals and granola bars. Cheerios has the highest content.[3]

Although Monsanto's marketing assures both farmer and consumer that these "traces" of weed killer are not harmful, it's also a highly profitable product. When you take into account the amount of cereals and other processed products you eat, the harm adds up, especially in children's growing bodies.

A wide variety of pesticides are used on commercially grown fruits and vegetables. The average strawberry has traces of thirteen different pesticides. That's why for the last five years, strawberries have topped the "dirty dozen" list of fruits and vegetables most contaminated with pesticides. Another list, the "clean fifteen" identifies foods that are still contaminated but have lower residue levels.[4]

The Dirty Dozen (commercially grown)

1. Strawberries
2. Spinach
3. Kale
4. Nectarines
5. Apples
6. Grapes*
7. Peaches
8. Cherries
9. Pears
10. Tomatoes
11. Celery
12. Potatoes

Raisins aren't officially on the list because they're considered a processed food, but they are just as contaminated as non-organic grapes. Ninety-nine percent of raisin samples tested revealed up to twenty-six different kinds of pesticides.

The Clean Fifteen (Commercially grown; fewer pesticides)

1. Avocado
2. Sweet corn*
3. Pineapple
4. Onion
5. Papaya*
6. Sweet peas (frozen)
7. Eggplant
8. Asparagus
9. Cauliflower
10. Cantaloupe
11. Broccoli
12. Mushroom
13. Cabbage
14. Honeydew melon
15. Kiwi

*Even with fewer pesticides, sweet corn and papaya can be grown from genetically modified seeds, so make sure they are non-GMO.

Switching to organic isn't just a fad. It's crucial to your long-term health. Everything you eat will be cleaner and more nutritious if it is organic. That includes spices, condiments, sweeteners, oils, vinegars—everything.

For the next twenty-one days, you will:

- Eat more plant-based foods and eliminate meat, eggs, dairy, processed food, junk food, and refined sugars from your diet.
- Stop drinking sodas, sports drinks, bottled fruit juices— anything but tea, water, and cold-pressed or homemade juices.
- Move your body every day. Walking is a wonderful way to start, especially if you are as out of shape as I was. If you're already exercising, you're ahead of the game. Keep it up!
- Journal what you eat and track your exercise.
- Talk to friends who support you.

- Not fall into the it's-only-one-day trap when eating out or attending a holiday or personal celebration.
- Cook more at home and eat out less. When you do eat out, you won't eat meat, eggs, or dairy products. No exceptions. Most restaurants now include plant-based dishes on their menus.

Author Lois McMaster Bujold said, "It's a bizarre but wonderful feeling to arrive dead center of a target you didn't even know you were aiming for." That's exactly the way I feel about my life today versus the way I was four years ago. You already know what you want.

On the following pages are tables listing your daily challenges. As you complete the challenge, check off the corresponding box. Don't beat yourself up if you slip up, but don't let yourself off the hook either. Remember procrastination and excuses are what led you here. Remember too, I am always on your side. You can do it.

TWENTY-ONE-DAY CHALLENGE							
DAYS 1 THROUGH 7 Check off each challenge when completed.	1	2	3	4	5	6	7
Eat a minimum of ONE plant-based meal a day.							
Drink only water, tea, or coffee. You can add plant milk to your coffee and fresh lemon or lime juice to your water and tea. If you use sweeteners, only use maple syrup or coconut sugar.							
Be mindful of what and why you eat. Feed your body, not your emotions.							
Enjoy a plant-based snack between meals. I don't mean potato chips. Check out the recipe section for ideas.							
Don't buy any highly processed foods. Read labels. Look for hidden sugar. Use the five-ingredient rule.							
Stop buying meat, eggs, and dairy products.							
When eating out, try a plant-based meal.							
Dump your junk food and don't eat fast food.							
Move for at least FIFTEEN minutes a day. Walk around your neighborhood, your backyard, or inside your home.							
Meditate for TEN minutes a day. You don't have to light candles and assume the lotus position. Sit quietly and look out the window. Use a free calming app. Daydream.							
Tell Inner Bitch to get lost every time you hear her voice.							
Add at least one self-supporting thought a day to your list.							
Track your food and exercise.							

TWENTY-ONE-DAY CHALLENGE							
DAYS 8 THROUGH 14 Check off each challenge when completed.	8	9	10	11	12	13	14
Eat a minimum of TWO plant-based meals a day.							
Drink only water, tea, or coffee. You can add plant milk to your coffee and fresh lemon or lime juice to your water and tea. If you use sweeteners, only use maple syrup or coconut sugar.							
Be mindful of what and why you eat. Feed your body, not your emotions.							
Enjoy a plant-based snack between meals.							
Don't buy highly-processed foods. Read labels. Look for hidden sugar. Use the five-ingredient rule.							
Don't buy meat, eggs, and dairy products.							
When eating out, eat ONLY plant-based dishes.							
If you still have junk food in the house, get rid of it now. Stay away from fast food.							
Move for at least TWENTY minutes a day. Walk around your neighborhood, your backyard, or inside your home.							
Meditate for TEN minutes a day.							
Keep telling Inner Bitch to shut the hell up.							
Add at least one self-supporting thought a day to your list.							
Track your food and exercise.							

TWENTY-ONE-DAY CHALLENGE							
DAYS 15 THROUGH 21 Check off each challenge when completed.	15	16	17	18	19	20	21
EAT NOTHING BUT PLANT-BASED MEALS!							
Drink only water, tea, or coffee. You can add plant milk to your coffee and fresh-squeezed lemon or lime juice to your water and tea. If you use sweeteners, only use maple syrup or coconut sugar.							
Be mindful of what and why you eat. Feed your body, not your emotions.							
ALL snacks should be plant-based.							
DON'T EAT ANY highly-processed foods. Read labels. Look for hidden sugar. Use the five-ingredient rule.							
DON'T EAT ANY meat, eggs, and dairy products.							
When eating out, eat ONLY plant-based dishes.							
Stay away from the junk food and fast food.							
Move for at least THIRTY minutes a day. Keep walking.							
Meditate for FIFTEEN minutes a day.							
Don't let Inner Bitch trick you with her best friend act. You've worked hard to get this far. Don't stop now.							
Add at least one self-supporting thought a day to your list.							
Track your food and exercise.							
CONGRATULATIONS! At the end of this week, give yourself a nonfood gift to celebrate!							

RECIPES

Our bodies are sophisticated biochemical machines that know how to extract the optimum nutrition from the foods we give it. Our brains are amazing biochemical computers that keep us alive. We don't need to think about breathing when we sleep. We don't need to think about how we digest our food or how to separate the nutrients in our foods. We have a built-in fight-or-flight instinct that warns us of danger. Except when it comes to what we eat.

Too often, we're like the proverbial frog in the pot of water that gradually heats up until it's boiled. Only our pot is full of sugar, artificial colors and flavors, pesticides, and a group of chemical preservatives too long to list. By the time we reach the boiling point, we have cancer, heart disease, diabetes, or any number of other diseases linked to poor diets and obesity. When you stop drugging yourself with the wrong foods, you give your body a chance to heal. All it needs from you is a healthy diet. I've included the following easy recipes to help you get started.

QUICK & EASY BREAKFASTS

Oatmeal Your Way

Fast and filling oatmeal will keep your body sated for hours. Eat it hot, or if your mornings are rushed, prepare overnight oats the night before.

Prep time: 10 minutes
Serves 2

Ingredients
1 cup whole grain, old-fashioned rolled oats
2 cups water
½ teaspoon cinnamon
Pinch of salt

Cook oats according to package directions. Divide into two bowls and add a splash of almond milk. Top with any of the following: ⅓ sliced banana, ½ cup frozen blueberries or strawberries, 1 teaspoon chopped walnuts, 1 teaspoon raisins or dried cranberries, or ½ chopped medium apple.

Too Rushed to Cook Oats

When you're cramped for time, make these the night before. You can either warm them up before you head out the door or take them with you for breakfast on the run.

Prep Time: 2 minutes
Serves 1

Ingredients
⅔ cup whole grain, old-fashioned rolled oats
2 teaspoons chia seeds (optional)
1 cup unsweetened almond milk
½ teaspoon cinnamon
¼ teaspoon nutmeg
1 teaspoon homemade vanilla (see recipe, page 153)
2 teaspoons maple syrup
Pinch of salt

In a container or jar with a tight lid, combine all of the ingredients. Stir everything together, tightly close the lid, and place in the refrigerator overnight.

Quick Quinoa Pancakes

Quinoa flour has a slightly nutty taste. This recipe is perfect if this is the first time you've tried it.

Prep time: 5 minutes
Cook time: 5–6 minutes
Makes 6–8 medium-size pancakes

Ingredients
1½ cups quinoa flour
½ cup unsweetened almond milk
½ cup unsweetened organic applesauce
1 teaspoon lemon juice
1 teaspoon baking soda
½ teaspoon homemade vanilla (optional) (see recipe, p. 153)
½ teaspoon cinnamon (optional)

In a large mixing bowl, stir all the ingredients together until the consistency of pancake batter. Don't overmix. Heat a twelve-inch nonstick pan that's been lightly sprayed with avocado oil over medium heat. Pour about a ¼ cup of batter into the pan for each pancake. Cook for two to three minutes on one side, then carefully flip and cook for another two to three minutes. Serve immediately with maple syrup.

Tip: Individual-size containers of applesauce are ideal for baking, so I keep a six-pack in the fridge. Each container is about a half cup, so there's no waste from a jar you might not finish using.

Protein-Packed Pancakes

Prep time: 5 minutes

Cook time: 5–6 minutes

Makes about 8–10 pancakes

Ingredients

2 scoops vanilla protein powder

1 cup whole grain, old-fashioned rolled oats

½ medium banana

1 cup unsweetened almond milk

1 teaspoon baking powder

Blend all ingredients in the blender until smooth. Lightly spray a nonstick frying pan with avocado oil and heat over medium heat. Pour about two tablespoons of batter into pan for each pancake. Cook for two minutes, or until top starts to bubble, and then flip and cook for about two more minutes until done. Serve with maple syrup.

Tip: Switch up this recipe by using chocolate protein powder. My favorite is Orgain Creamy Chocolate Fudge.

SMOOTHIES

Although I've put these recipes in the breakfast section, there's almost no end to the variety of nutritious and delicious smoothies you can make. Green smoothies are satisfying for either breakfast or lunch. You can add a handful of spinach to any fruit smoothie. You can add protein powder for an extra boost of nutrition or simply have them with almost any combination of fruits, nut milk, and flavorings. All smoothie recipes are one serving.

Double Vanilla Protein Smoothie

Ingredients

1 cup unsweetened almond milk
2 scoops vanilla protein powder
½ medium banana, sliced
½ teaspoon cinnamon
1 teaspoon homemade vanilla (see recipe, page 153)
1 cup ice

Pour the almond milk into a blender. Add the protein powder, cinnamon, and vanilla and blend until smooth. Add the banana and ice and blend. If the mix is too thin, add more ice. If too frozen, add a little water.

Tip #1: I use Orgain Vanilla Bean protein powder. It has twenty-one grams of protein per serving and is all organic, vegan, soy-free, and inexpensive.

Tip #2: Buy extra bananas and then peel, cut in half, and freeze them.

Fast and Fruity Smoothie

Ingredients

1 cup unsweetened almond milk

1 small banana, sliced

1 cup frozen fruit of your choice

(blueberry, strawberry, pineapple, mango, or a mixed blend)

1–2 tablespoons chia seeds (optional)

½ teaspoon grated fresh ginger or 1 teaspoon ground ginger

Toss everything in the blender and blend until smooth.

Green Power Smoothie

Ingredients

1 cup unsweetened almond milk

1 cup fresh baby spinach, washed and patted dry

1 large frozen banana, sliced into 1-inch pieces

1 tablespoon chia seeds

1 tablespoon organic peanut or almond butter

1 cup ice

Mix everything in blender and enjoy.

INTERCHANGEABLE LUNCH & DINNERS

CONTAINER SALADS

These fresh salads are full of flavor. Carrots, apples, mixed greens, red cabbage, green or red onions, corn, avocado, black or white beans, and grape tomatoes are just a few of the vegetables and fruits you can use. You can add raisins, dried cranberries, sunflower seeds, peanuts, pecans, quinoa, and rice.

Layer like this: Dressing on the bottom, hard vegetables and fruit next, wet vegetables (cucumber/tomato) and grains next, and greens and nuts last. Mix together just before eating.

Santa Fe Salad with Quinoa & Cilantro-Lime Dressing

Prep time: 20 minutes
Cook time: 15 minutes
Makes 4 salads

Ingredients
1 15-ounce can black beans, drained and rinsed
1 cup frozen corn, thawed
1 cup grape tomatoes, halved
1 small red bell pepper, chopped
1 small green bell pepper, chopped
3 green onions, sliced
1 medium avocado, diced

Quinoa
1 cup quinoa
2 cups water

Combine quinoa and water in a quart saucepan. Bring to boil, and then reduce to a simmer. Cover and cook for fifteen minutes or until all the water is absorbed. Remove from heat and let stand for five minutes, and then uncover and let cool completely.

Cilantro-Lime Dressing

Make the dressing while the quinoa cooks.

1 cup fresh cilantro

2 teaspoons cumin

2 garlic cloves

½ cup lime juice (about 3 to 4 limes)

½ teaspoon chili powder

1 tablespoon extra-virgin olive oil

Pinch of salt

Put all ingredients in the blender and blend until smooth.

Divide the dressing between four containers. Next, layer the black beans, corn, cooled quinoa, bell peppers, green onion, tomatoes, and avocado. Seal the containers and put in the refrigerator.

Tip: Here's where your frozen herbs can come in handy. Use four frozen cubes or a cup of frozen leaves.

Asian Crunch Salad with Peanut Dressing

In one evening, you can make lunch for the week ahead. These layered salads will keep in the refrigerator for up to five days. Container salads are a great way to get your kids involved in creating healthy lunches to take to school. You'll need BPA-free plastic containers with air-tight lids, forks or spoons, and napkins.

Ingredients

1 cup shredded red cabbage

½ cup unsalted peanuts, chopped

1 cup shredded carrots

1 cup broccoli florets, chopped

¾ cup cauliflower florets, chopped

¾ cup red bell pepper, diced

2 green onions, sliced

2 cups romaine, torn

Peanut Dressing

1 tablespoon creamy peanut butter

1 tablespoon Bragg's liquid aminos

½ teaspoon hot sauce (I use Sriracha.)

Mix well.

Divide the dressing between four containers. Next, layer the broccoli, cauliflower, cabbage, carrots, bell pepper, romaine, green onions, and peanuts. Seal the containers and put in the refrigerator.

Chickpea Wraps

Prep time: 10 minutes

Serves 4

Ingredients

1 15-ounce can chickpeas (garbanzo beans),
      rinsed and drained

½ cup celery, chopped

½ cup red onion, chopped

½ kosher dill pickle, finely chopped

Juice from 1 medium or ½ large lemon

¼ cup vegan mayonnaise (I use Vegenaise Soy-Free)

1 teaspoon garlic powder

1 teaspoon Bragg's Organic Sprinkle

½ teaspoon dried basil, crushed

1 tablespoon Old Bay seasoning

½ teaspoon black pepper

4 large romaine lettuce leaves, washed and patted dry

In a large bowl, mash chickpeas with a fork until broken into small pieces. Add the rest of the ingredients and mix well. Divide evenly between the romaine leaves and roll up.

Pantry Chili

Prep time: 10 minutes
Cook time: 20 minutes
Serves 6

Ingredients

1 15-ounce can black beans, drained and rinsed
1 15-ounce can pinto beans, drained and rinsed
1 15-ounce can Great Northern beans, drained and rinsed
1 14.5-ounce can chopped tomatoes
1 4-ounce can fire-roasted diced green chilies
    (Optional. You choose the heat level.)
½ cup red wine
¾ cup corn, frozen (optional)
1 medium yellow onion, chopped
1 small green bell pepper, chopped
4 teaspoons red chili powder
1 teaspoon garlic powder
1 teaspoon ground cumin
1 teaspoon oregano leaves, crushed
1 teaspoon basil leaves, crushed
2 teaspoons coconut sugar
½ teaspoon salt
½ teaspoon black pepper
Olive oil cooking spray
Optional garnishes: chopped green onions, cilantro,
    and a squeeze of lime

Spray the bottom and sides of a six-quart saucepan with olive oil and sauté the onion and bell pepper until translucent. Then add the spices and stir for about a minute to release their oils. Add the remaining ingredients, stir well, and bring to a boil. Reduce heat and simmer for twenty-five minutes, stirring occasionally. You can add Sriracha or your favorite hot sauce to taste.

Tip: Keep a four-pack of the 6-ounce bottles of red and white wines in the pantry. That's a little more than a half cup, but the extra will keep in the fridge. Or you can use it in the chili for a deeper flavor.

Roasted Vegetable Tacos

Prep time: 10 minutes

Cook time: 25 minutes

Makes 10 tacos

Ingredients

1 large white or yellow onion, cut into 1-inch cubes

2 cups cauliflower florets

3 red potatoes, cut into 1-inch cubes

1 medium bell pepper, cut into ½-inch strips

½ teaspoon cumin

1 teaspoon chili powder

3 cloves of garlic, minced

½ teaspoon salt

Olive oil cooking spray

10 corn tortillas (non-GMO)

Optional garnishes: Avocado, lime juice, cilantro,
     thinly sliced radishes, and pepitas

Preheat oven to 375°. Arrange vegetables on a nonstick baking sheet and spray lightly with olive oil. Mix cumin, chili powder, garlic, and salt together and sprinkle over vegetables. Gently toss vegetables to combine, spread in an even layer, and bake for twenty minutes.

Remove tortillas from package and arrange in an oven-proof dish. Place in the oven to warm during the last five minutes the vegetables are roasting. To serve, fill each taco with the roasted vegetables and garnishes. Top with your favorite fresh or jarred organic salsa.

Ginger-Carrot Bisque

Prep time: 10 minutes
Cook time: 15 minutes
Serves 4

Ingredients

2 cups low-sodium vegetable broth
1 13-ounce can unsweetened coconut milk
2 teaspoons curry powder
1 tablespoon fresh ginger, grated
1 cup yellow onion, chopped
2 cups fresh carrots, peeled and chopped
2 garlic cloves, minced
½ teaspoon sea salt
1 tablespoon fresh lime juice
Fresh chopped chives for garnish

In a two-quart saucepan, combine vegetable broth, ginger, curry powder, carrots, onion, and garlic. Bring to boil, cover, and reduce heat. Simmer until carrots are tender, about ten minutes. Remove from heat and blend with immersion blender until consistency of a puree. Add salt, lime juice, and coconut milk. Stir to blend. Return to heat if needed to increase temperature. Spoon into soup bowls and garnish with chives.

EXTRAS

Dill Sauce

Use this sauce for a salad dressing, a dip for vegetables, or on a baked potato.

Prep time: 3 minutes
Makes 1 cup

Ingredients
¾ cup vegan mayonnaise (I use Vegenaise Soy-Free.)
1–2 teaspoons lime juice, fresh-squeezed
1 teaspoon dill weed, crushed
1 teaspoon red onion, minced (optional)
¼ teaspoon salt

Mix all ingredients together until they are a creamy consistency. If too thick, add more lime juice. Adjust seasonings to taste. Will keep in the refrigerator for up to three days.

Easy Vinaigrette Dressing

Ingredients

⅓ cup Bragg's Organic Apple Cider Vinegar

2 teaspoons maple syrup

1½ teaspoons Dijon mustard

2 cloves garlic, crushed

1 teaspoon dried oregano, crushed

½ teaspoon sea salt

¼ cup olive or avocado oil

Fresh ground black pepper

You can either blend the ingredients in a blender, whisk together in a small bowl, or put in a jar and shake. Adjust the seasonings to your taste. Dressing will keep up to five days in the refrigerator.

Homemade Hummus

Prep time: 5 minutes

Makes 1 cup

Ingredients

1 15-ounce can chickpeas (garbanzo beans),
    rinsed and drained

2 cloves garlic

½ teaspoon cumin

Juice of 1–2 lemons, to taste

2–3 tablespoons water for consistency

½ teaspoon sea salt

Toss all ingredients in a food processor and blend to the desired consistency. Adjust the seasonings to your taste. Serve with carrot sticks, bell pepper slices, apple slices, or torn pita bread.

Homemade Vanilla Extract in the Instant Pot

Prep time: 15 minutes
Cook time: 45 minutes
Rest time to let pressure return to normal: 30 minutes
Makes 16 oz.

Ingredients
16 ounces rum
10 Grade A or B vanilla beans
1 cup water

Wash and dry two eight-ounce Mason jars and lids. Pour 1 cup of rum into each jar. Slit the vanilla beans to release their oil. Place five beans in each jar. Screw the lids on the jars just until fingertip tight. Don't over-tighten or they could explode inside the cooker.

Put the steamer rack in the pot of the cooker and pour in the water. Sit the jars on the middle of the rack. Close the lid, seal the valve, and cook on manual high pressure for forty-five minutes. Let steam naturally release—about thirty minutes. Use oven gloves to remove the jars, and a towel to tighten the lids. Don't remove the beans.

Store in a dark place (like the back of the pantry) at room temperature. Let the extract's flavor develop for a minimum of forty-eight hours. A couple of weeks is even better.

Recommended Resources

I encourage you to investigate and experiment with more plant-based foods. Here are a few of my favorite sites to help you get started.

- A Couple Cooks, https://www.acouplecooks.com/about/
- Assuaged, https://www.assuaged.com/
- Connoisseurus Veg, https://www.connoisseurusveg.com/
- Forks Over Knives, https://www.forksoverknives.com/our-story/
- *Olive Magazine*, https://www.olivemagazine.com/recipes/vegan/healthy-vegan-recipes-under-350-calories/
- Vegansandra, http://www.vegansandra.com/2017/06/15-delicious-vegan-recipes-for-beginners.html
- Yum Vegan Food, https://yumveganlunchideas.com/the-best-low-calorie-vegan-recipes/

ENDNOTES

INTRODUCTION

1 "People with Certain Medical Conditions," Center for Disease Control and Prevention, https://www.cdc.gov/coronavirus/2019-ncov/need-extra-precautions/people -with-medical-conditions.html.

2 Lisa M. Nackers, Kathryn M. Ross, and Michael G. Perri, "The Association Between Rate of Initial Weight Loss and Long-Term Success in Obesity Treatment: Does Slow and Steady Win the Race?" *International Journal of Behavioral Medicine* 17, no. 3 (2010): 161–167, https://doi.org/10.1007/s12529-010-9092-y.

3 Harriet Brown, "The Weight of the Evidence," Slate, March 24, 2015, https:// slate.com/technology/2015/03/diets-do-not-work-the-thin-evidence-that-losing- weight-makes-you-healthier.html.

CHAPTER 2

1 Michaela Kiernan, et al., "Social support for healthy behaviors: Scale psychometrics and prediction of weight loss among women in a behavioral program," *Obesity* 20, no. 4 (2012): 756–764, https://doi.org/10.1038/oby.2011.293.

CHAPTER 3

1 "Jon Kabat-Zinn: Defining Mindfulness," *Mindful*, January 11, 2017, https://www. mindful.org/jon-kabat-zinn-defining-mindfulness/.

2 Lisa Firestone, PhD, "4 Ways to Overcome Your Inner Critic," *Psychology Today*, May 14, 2013, https://www.psychologytoday.com/us/blog/compassion-matters/201305 /4-ways-overcome-your-inner-critic.

3 Michelle May, MD, "Reprogram Your Brain," *Huffington Post*, June 20, 2014, updated December 6, 2017, https://www.huffpost.com/entry/reprogram-your-brain _b_5515443.

4 Kris Hallbom and Tim Hallbom, "Neuroscience & Creating an Optimal Future for Yourself," The NLP Institute of California, August 12, 2012, https://nlpca.com/ creating-an-optimal-future-for-yourself/.

CHAPTER 5

1 Albrecht Powell, "Top 10 New Year's Resolutions," liveabout.com, updated June 19, 2020, https://www.liveabout.com/popular-new-years-resolutions-2708154; Shainna Ali, PhD, LMHC, "Why New Year's Resolutions Fail," *Psychology Today*, December 5, 2018, https://www.psychologytoday.com/us/blog/modern-mentality/201812/why-new-years-resolutions-fail.

CHAPTER 6

1 "Wedding weight loss: Survey finds only 18 percent of brides hit their target weight before the big day," Toronto.com, August 26, 2019, https://www.toronto.com/community-story/9560144-wedding-weight-loss-survey-finds-only-18-per-cent-of-brides-hit-their-target-weight-before-the-big-day/.

2 "SlimFast Advanced Nutrition Creamy Chocolate Shake – Ready to Drink Meal –20g of Protein," Amazon, https://www.amazon.com/SlimFast-Advanced-Nutrition-Creamy-Chocolate/dp/B0187HZG2E.

3 "SlimFast Keto Fat Bomb Snacks, Peanut Butter Cup," Amazon, https://www.amazon.com/SlimFast-Snacks-Peanut-Butter-Grams/dp/B07H7NPY5D/ref=sr_1_4?crid=3KLJTMGA1MVE3&dchild=1&keywords=slim+fast+-fat+bombs&qid=1594319284&s=hpc&sprefix=slim+fast+fat+bomb%2Chpc%2C232&sr=1-4.

4 "Slim-Fast Foods Company History," FundingUniverse, http://www.fundinguniverse.com/company-histories/slim-fast-foods-company-history/.

5 "48 Hour Miracle Diet®," Hollywood Diet, https://hollywooddiet.com/48-hour-miracle-diet.html.

6 "LA Lites—Nutrition Bar," My Fitness Pal, https://www.myfitnesspal.com/food/calories/nutrition-bar-919059; "How much sugar is too much?" American Heart Association, https://www.heart.org/en/healthy-living/healthy-eating/eat-smart/sugar/how-much-sugar-is-too-much.

CHAPTER 7

1 Becky Little, "When Cigarette Companies Used Doctors to Push Smoking," *History*, September 13, 2018, updated September 11, 2019, https://www.history.com/news/cigarette-ads-doctors-smoking-endorsement.

2 Lucky Strike Cigarettes, "When Tempted Reach for a Lucky Instead," Print advertisement, 1930, http://tobacco.stanford.edu/tobacco_main/images.php?token2=fm_st046.php&token1=fm_img1138.php&theme_file=fm_mt014.php&theme_name=Keeps

3 "How Magician Penn Jillette Lost 100 Pounds on Potato Diet," *Houston Chronicle*, June 19, 2019, https://www.chron.com/news/article/How-magician-Penn-Jillette-lost-100-pounds-on-14019288.php.

4 Ibid.

ENDNOTES

5   Ibid.

6   Ernie Smith, "Giving Candy a Bad Name," Tedium, September 20, 2018, https://tedium.co/2018/09/20/ayds-candy-branding-problem/.

7   Ibid.

8   "History of the REAL Dr. Siegal's COOKIE DIET®," Dr. Siegal's Cookie Diet, https://www.cookiediet.com/about-us/cookie-history/.

9   "How to Use the Hollywood Diet," Hollywood Diet, https://hollywooddiet.com/how-to-use-the-hollywood-diet; "Chocolate Chip Cookies," https://hollywooddiet.com/hollywood-diet-products/the-hollywood-cookie-diet-chocolate-chip.html.

10 Michael Dhar, "What is Jell-O?" Live Science, December 19, 2013, https://www.livescience.com/42088-what-is-jello-jell-o.html.

11 "Super Fat Burning Gummies," SkinnyMint, https://www.skinnymint.com/products/super-fat-burning-gummies-2-step-bundle?gclid=EAIaIQobChMIh4yGktTI6gIVBdvACh1OnwBHEAAYASAAEgKOEvD_BwE.

12 Judith Weinraub, "The Cabbage Soup Diet," The Washington Post, February 21, 1996, https://www.washingtonpost.com/archive/lifestyle/food/1996/02/21/the-cabbage-soup-diet/25081d4f-ebd4-4c48-ba7e-a6d7af4edb54/.

13 Marvo, "Fast Food Flashback: McDonald's McLean Deluxe," The Impulsive Buy, March 7, 2015, https://www.theimpulsivebuy.com/wordpress/2015/03/07/fast-food-flashback-mcdonalds-mclean-deluxe/.

14 "How alli® Works," Alli, https://www.myalli.com/about/how-alli-works/; "Xenical," Rx List, updated May 20, 2020, https://www.rxlist.com/xenical-drug.htm.

15 "Gloria Marshall Figure Salon Equipment," Google, https://www.google.com/search?sa=X&source=univ&tbm=isch&q=gloria+marshall+figure+salon+equipment&ved=2ahUKEwjs4NaVkMnqAhUCNKwKHQ0aB3EQsAR6BAgJEAE&biw=1229&bih=579.

16 "Best Sellers in Vibration Platform Machines," Amazon, https://www.amazon.com/Best-Sellers-Sports-Outdoors-Vibration-Platform-Machines/zgbs/sporting-goods/1297872011; Powerfit Elite, https://www.powerfitelite.com/?utm_source=google&utm_medium=shopping&gclid=EAIaIQobChMIire075HJ6gIVzM-DACh20WAM9EAQYASABEgKPqPD_BwE.

17 Edward R. Laskowski, M.D., "Is whole-body vibration a good way to lose weight and improve fitness?" Mayo Clinic, April 8, 2020, https://www.mayoclinic.org/healthy-lifestyle/fitness/expert-answers/whole-body-vibration/faq-20057958.

18 "'Wonder Sauna Hot Pants' Was the Most '70s Product to Hit the Market," MeTV, March 14, 2016, https://www.metv.com/stories/wonder-sauna-hot-pants-was-the-most-70s-product-to-hit-the-market.

19 "Obesity: Facts, Figures, Guidelines," West Virginia Department of Health and Human Resources, December 2002, https://www.wvdhhr.org/bph/oehp/obesity/mortality.htm.

20 Liam Davenport and Lisa Nainggolan, "Obesity link to severe COVID-19, especially in patients under 60," *The Hospitalist*, April 17, 2020, https://www.the-hospitalist.org/hospitalist/article/220925/obesity/obesity-link-severe-covid-19-especially-patients-aged-under-60.

21 Mandy Oaklander, "Here's How Many Calories You'll Eat During the Super Bowl," *TIME*, January 29, 2015, https://time.com/3687510/super-bowl-snacks-calories/.

CHAPTER 8

1 Harriet Brown, "The Weight of the Evidence," Slate, March 24, 2015, https://slate.com/technology/2015/03/diets-do-not-work-the-thin-evidence-that-losing-weight-makes-you-healthier.html.

2 "Weight Watchers Revenue: How Does Weight Watchers Make Money?," Trefis, August 20, 2019, https://dashboards.trefis.com/no-login-required/AFAUNzz4/Weight-Watchers-Revenue%3A-How-Does-Weight-Watchers-Make-Money%3F; "Nutrisystem Announces Fourth Quarter and Full Year 2018 Financial Results," *Business Wire*, February 19, 2019, https://www.businesswire.com/news/home/20190219005700/en/Nutrisystem-Announces-Fourth-Quarter-Full-Year-2018; Jaewon Kang and Lillian Rizzo, "Jenny Craig Weighs Sale as Performance Improves," *Wall Street Journal*, updated September 12, 2018, https://www.wsj.com/articles/jenny-craig-weighs-a-sale-after-bulking-up-balance-sheet-1536748200.

3 "Introducing My WW," Weight Watchers, https://www.weightwatchers.com/us/how-it-works.

4 Traci Mann, "Oprah's Investment in Weight Watchers Was Smart Because the Program Doesn't Work," Slate, November 3, 2015, https://slate.com/culture/2015/11/why-weight-watchers-doesn-t-work.html.

5 "ZeroPoint Cheat Sheet: Fruit," Weight Watchers, https://www.weightwatchers.com/us/article/zero-points-cheat-sheet-fruit.

6 Lora E. Burke, Jing Wang, and Mary Ann Sevick, "Self-Monitoring in Weight Loss: A Systematic Review of the Literature," *Journal of the American Dietetic Association* 111, no. 1 (2011): 92–102, https://doi.org/10.1016/j.jada.2010.10.008.

7 Jelisa Castrodale, "Weight Watchers Under Fire for Diet and Food Tracking App for Kids," *Vice*, August 16, 2019, https://www.vice.com/en_us/article/pa7d4g/weight-watchers-under-fire-for-diet-and-food-tracking-app-for-kids.

8 Miranda Hitti, "Lasting Damage from Fen-Phen Drug?" WebMD, November 5, 2008, https://www.webmd.com/heart-disease/news/20081105/lasting-heart-damage-from-fen-phen#.

9 Luisa Yanez, "Nutri/System Settles Local Lawsuits," *South Florida Sun Sentinel*, November 7, 1991, http://articles.sun-sentinel.com/1991-11-07/news/9102150288_1_nutri-gallbladder-disease-rapid-weight; Lauren Silvis, summarized by Heather Salazar, "Nutrisystem: Gallbladder Problems Due to Diet (1991)," Business Ethics Case Analyses, December 30, 2012, http://businessethicscases.blogspot.

com/2012/12/case-nutrisystem-consumers-gallbladders_30.html; David Kinney, "National diet center chain pulls fen-phen,"*Associated Press*, September 3, 1997, https://apnews.com/b6bc748a872e912b23a45afd7297b890.

10 "Nutrisystem Turbo Chocolate Shake Mix, 1.4 Oz, 20 Packets," Walmart, https://www.walmart.com/ip/Nutrisystem-Turbo-Chocolate-Shake-Mix-1-4-Oz-20-Packets/277626113.

11 "Jenny Craig, Inc. History," FundingUniverse, http://www.fundinguniverse.com/company-histories/jenny-craig-inc-history/.

12 "Jenny Craig, Inc. History," FundingUniverse, http://www.fundinguniverse.com/company-histories/jenny-craig-inc-history/.

13 Hanae Armitage, "Low-fat or low-carb? It's a draw, study finds," Stanford Medicine News Center, February 20, 2018, https://med.stanford.edu/news/all-news/2018/02/low-fat-or-low-carb-its-a-draw-study-finds.html.

14 Gretchen Voss, "When You Lose Weight—And Gain It All Back," *Women's Health*, June 6, 2010, http://www.nbcnews.com/id/36716808/ns/health-diet_and_nutrition/t/when-you-lose-weight-gain-it-all-back/#.X1B4TtVKipo.

15 Raphael Chestang, "Valerie Bertinelli Talks Ditching the Scale After 40-Pound Weight Loss," *Entertainment Tonight*, August 6, 2015, https://www.etonline.com/news/169497_valerie_bertinelli_talks_ditching_the_scale_after_40_pound_weight_loss.

CHAPTER 9

1 Nicolas Rasmussen, PhD, MPhil, MPH, "America's First Amphetamine Epidemic 1929–1971," *American Journal of Public Health* 98, no. 6 (2008): 974–985, https://doi.org/10.2105/AJPH.2007.110593.

2 Ibid.

3 N.R. Kleinfield, "Just What Killed the Diet Doctor, And What Keeps the Issue Alive?," *The New York Times*, February 11, 2004, https://www.nytimes.com/2004/02/11/nyregion/just-what-killed-the-diet-doctor-and-what-keeps-the-issue-alive.html.

4 "Creating Health for Your Patients and Your Practice," Optavia, https://www.optavia.com/health-coaching-opportunities/health-professional.

5 "Weight regain after bariatric surgery," Mayo Clinic, June 13, 2018, https://www.mayoclinic.org/medical-professionals/endocrinology/news/weight-regain-after-bariatric-surgery/mac-20431467.

6 "Plant-Based Diet Reverses Heart Disease," Physicians Committee for Responsible Medicine, July 1, 2014, https://www.pcrm.org/news/health-nutrition/plant-based-diet-reverses-heart-disease.

7 Rachel Cernansky, "Your doctor may not be the best source of nutrition advice," *The Washington Post*, July 8, 2018, https://www.washingtonpost.com/national/health-science/your-doctor-may-not-be-the-best-source-of-nutrition-advice/2018/07/06/f8b3ecfe-78af-11e8-93cc-6d3beccdd7a3_story.html

8 Katherine Gergen Barnett, MD, "Physician Obesity: The Tipping Point," *Global Advances in Health and Medicine* 3, no. 6 (2014): 8-10, https://doi.org/10.7453/gahmj.2014.061.

9 "Chocolate Ice Crush Shake Mix," South Beach Diet, https://www.southbeachdiet.com/diet-nutrition/5133/snacks/90153/chocolate+ice+crush+shake+mix.

10 "Heart Disease in the United States," Centers for Disease Control and Prevention, June 22, 2020, https://www.cdc.gov/heartdisease/facts.html; "Heart Disease and Stroke Cost America Nearly $1 Billion a Day in Medical Costs, Lost Productivity," CDC Foundation, April 29, 2015, https://www.cdcfoundation.org/pr/2015/heart-disease-and-stroke-cost-america-nearly-1-billion-day-medical-costs-lost-productivity; Benjamin Baddeley, Sangeetha Sornalingam, and Max Cooper, "Sitting is the new smoking: where do we stand?" *British Journal of Medical Practice* 66, no. 646 (2016): 258, https://doi.org/10.3399/bjgp16X685009.

CHAPTER 10

1 "80% of Celebrity Endorsed Foods Are Unhealthy," *Longevity*, June 2016, https://www.longevitylive.com/editors-choice/80-celebrity-endorsed-foods-unhealthy/.

2 "Adult Obesity Facts," Centers for Disease Control and Prevention, https://www.cdc.gov/obesity/data/adult.html.

3 "The 28 Worst Breakfast Cereals—Ranked!," Eat This, Not That!, November 30, 2015, https://www.eatthis.com/worst-breakfast-cereals/.

4 Gloria M. Reeves, MD, Teodor T. Postolache, MD, and Soren Snitker, MD, PhD, "Childhood Obesity and Depression: Connection between these Growing Problems in Growing Children," *International Journal of Child Health and Human Development* 1, no. 2 (2008): 103-114, https://www.ncbi.nlm.nih.gov/pmc/articles/PMC2568994/.

5 Grace Chen, "Why Fast Food is 'Healthier' Than School Lunches: The Shocking USDA Truth," Public School Review, updated May 21, 2020, https://www.publicschoolreview.com/blog/why-fast-food-is-healthier-than-school-lunches-the-shocking-usda-truth.

CHAPTER 11

1 A. Pawlowski, "Half of Americans are trying to lose weight: 8 tips for lasting success," Today, July 12, 2018, https://www.today.com/health/dieting-lose-weight-half-americans-trying-slim-down-t133099.

2 Bob Greene, "Oprah's Weight Loss Confession," Oprah.com, January 5, 2009, https://www.oprah.com/health/oprahs-weight-loss-confession/all.

3 Nicole Avena, "How Sugar Affects the Brain," TEDEd, https://ed.ted.com/lessons/how-sugar-affects-the-brain-nicole-avena.

4 Matt Nelson, "Refined Tastes: Are Some Foods Addictive?," *University of Michigan News*, January 18, 2019, https://rackham.umich.edu/discover-rackham/refined-tastes-are-some-food-addictive/.

5   Magalie Lenoir, Fuschia Serre, Lauriane Cantin, and Serge H. Ahmed, "Intense Sweetness Surpasses Cocaine Reward," *PLoS One* 2, no. 8 (2007), https://doi.org/10.1371/journal.pone.0000698.
6   Eliza L. Gordon, Aviva H. Ariel-Donges, Viviana Bauman, and Lisa J. Merlo, "What is the Evidence for 'Food Addiction?' A Systematic Review," *Nutrients* 10, no. 4 (2018): 477, https://www.ncbi.nlm.nih.gov/pmc/articles/PMC5946262/.
7   "Food Addiction," WebMD, updated July 17, 2020, https://www.webmd.com/mental-health/eating-disorders/binge-eating-disorder/mental-health-food-addiction#1.

CHAPTER 12
1   "Obesity and Overweight," Centers for Disease Control and Prevention, updated February 28, 2020, https://www.cdc.gov/nchs/fastats/obesity-overweight.htm.
2   Raffi Khatchadourian, "The Taste Makers," *The New Yorker*, November 23, 2009, https://www.newyorker.com/magazine/2009/11/23/the-taste-makers.
3   Kristen Fischer, "Is Red Dye 40 Toxic?" Healthline, April 2, 2015, updated September 17, 2018, https://www.healthline.com/health/food-nutrition/is-red-dye-40-toxic%23overview1.
4   "Sodium in Your Diet," U.S. Food and Drug Administration, April 2, 2020, https://www.fda.gov/food/nutrition-education-resources-materials/sodium-your-diet; "Added Sugar in the Diet," T.H. Chan School of Public Health, Harvard, https://www.hsph.harvard.edu/nutritionsource/carbohydrates/added-sugar-in-the-diet/.
5   "45 Alarming Statistics on American's [*sic*] Sugar Consumption and the Effects of Sugar on Americans' Health," TheDiabetesCouncil.com, July 10, 2018, https://www.thediabetescouncil.com/45-alarming-statistics-on-americans-sugar-consumption-and-the-effects-of-sugar-on-americans-health/.
6   "Type 2 Diabetes in Children," Healthline, March 7, 2019, https://www.healthline.com/health/type-2-diabetes-children.
7   "Bush's Vegetarian Baked Beans – 16 oz," Amazon, https://www.amazon.com/Bushs-Vegetarian-Baked-Beans-16/dp/B0005Z7F2Q.
8   Ashley Welch, "Do you know how much sugar is in your Starbucks drink?," CBS News, February 19, 2016, https://www.cbsnews.com/news/do-you-know-how-much-sugar-is-in-your-starbucks-drink/.
9   Kathryn Watson, "Type 3 Diabetes and Alzheimer's Disease: What You Need to Know," Healthline, June 28, 2018, https://www.healthline.com/health/type-3-diabetes#diagnosis.
10 Paul K. Crane, MD, MPH, et al, "Glucose Levels and Risk of Dementia," *New England Journal of Medicine* 369 (2013): 540–548, https://doi.org/10.1056/NEJMoa1215740/.
11 "Added Sugars," American Heart Association, updated April 17, 2018, https://www.heart.org/en/healthy-living/healthy-eating/eat-smart/sugar/added-sugars; "How

Much Sugar Is Too Much?" American Heart Association, https://www.heart.org/en/healthy-living/healthy-eating/eat-smart/sugar/how-much-sugar-is-too-much.

12 Mandy Oaklander, "Soda May Age You as Much as Smoking, Study Says," *TIME*, October 17, 2014, https://time.com/3513875/soda-may-age-you-as-much-as-smoking/.

13 "How Much Sugar Is in Coca-cola?," Coca-cola Company, https://www.coca-colacompany.com/faqs/how-much-sugar-is-in-coca-cola; Joe Leech, "13 Ways That Sugary Soda Is Bad for Your Health," Healthline, February 8, 2019, https://www.healthline.com/nutrition/13-ways-sugary-soda-is-bad-for-you#section4.

CHAPTER 13

1 Chris K. Guerin, MD, FNLA, FAC, and Rajasreepai Ramachandra Pai, MD, "The Argument for Plant-Based Diets," *Empower Magazine*, Vol 9 Issue 2, https://www.empoweryourhealth.org/magazine/vol9_issue2/the_argument_for_plant_based_diets.

2 Cecelia Smith-Schoenwalder, "What to Know About Glyphosate, the Pesticide in Roundup Weed Killer," *U.S. News*, August 19, 2019, https://www.usnews.com/news/national-news/articles/what-to-know-about-glyphosate-the-pesticide-in-roundup-weed-killer.

3 Alexa Lardieri, "Cancer-Causing Ingredient in Weedkiller Found in Cheerios," *U.S. News*, June 12, 2019, https://www.usnews.com/news/health-news/articles/2019-06-12/cancer-causing-ingredient-in-roundup-weedkiller-found-in-cheerios-nature-valley-products.

4 "Dirty Dozen: EWG's 2020 Shopper's Guide to Pesticides in Produce," Environmental Working Group, https://www.ewg.org/foodnews/dirty-dozen.php; "Clean Fifteen: EWG's 2020 Shopper's Guide to Pesticides in Produce," Environmental Working Group, https://www.ewg.org/foodnews/clean-fifteen.php.

ACKNOWLEDGMENTS

Although writing is a solitary profession, no one writes a book alone. Thank you to Bonnie Hearn Hill who has been beside me since my first stumbling step back to health, and who set the example of health and plant-based living that I've tried to follow; to Stacy Renee Lucas for always coming up with the right words in the right places, and patiently reading and re-reading every chapter of this book; and to my daughter, Wendy Cooper, for supporting me in every way, every day.

Grateful thanks to Anthony Ziccardi, Maddie Sturgeon, Devon Brown, and the team at Post Hill Press for helping to make my book a reality.

ABOUT THE AUTHOR

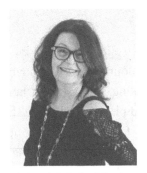

Author photo by Derek Lapsley

Hazel Dixon-Cooper, once described by a book reviewer as, "...funnier and franker than your best friend after three drinks," spent almost nine years advising the readers of *Cosmopolitan* magazine about love, money, life, and astrology. Yet, she couldn't fix her own life. Now, after losing and keeping off 122 pounds, along with considerable emotional baggage, she is an integrative nutrition health/wellness coach and author committed to helping others change their lives.